FOOD ALLERGY GUIDE

TO SOY

HOW TO EAT
SAFELY AND WELL

SOY-FREE

BILL BOWLING

FOOD ALLERGY GUIDE TO

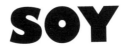

HOW TO EAT SAFELY AND WELL SOY-FREE

BILL BOWLING

RIDGELINE PUBLISHING
Frankfort, Kentucky

Food Allergy Guide to Soy:
How to Eat Safely and Well Soy-Free
Bill Bowling

Copyright © 2014 (Bill Bowling)

Contact Information:
billbowlinginformation@gmail.com
http://billbowling.weebly.com
http://ridgelinepublishing.weebly.com

ISBN: 978-0-9834571-3-8
ISBN/e-reader: 978-0-9834571-5-2

Printed in the United States of America

Book Design by Bill Bowling
Cover Design by Anahlisha Bowling

First Edition: June, 2014

DEDICATION

To

Katrina, my wife, who has cooked her way deliciously out of soy allergy hell.

"The greatest wealth is health."
–Unknown

"To eat is a necessity, but to eat intelligently is an art."
— François de La Rochefoucauld

ACKNOWLEDGMENTS/NOTES

Although writing appears to be a solitary process, it isn't. Besides the precious time poured into any project, there is much invaluable help and input along the way that any writer takes for granted to his or her own detriment. There is of course much more to it than the chiseling of words into a stone slab—that's the end result, and it is work, don't get me wrong: There's the mountain of reading material; there's the talking and the learning; there's the digging for and sorting out of strands of information; there's the organizing; there's the fact checking; there's the editing and proofing; there's the designing so that the finished product is something you can be proud of, something that you can stand behind with surety and confidence.

There are many thanks and grateful nods that must be extended in any circumstance of authorship, and here is no different. Let me get started with this very happy task by first and foremost acknowledging my wife, Katrina, who shared freely all she has learned in dealing with a soy allergy. She is the catalyst for the book, and she is proof positive that an allergen can be conquered and that a sufferer can live and eat well. Her input was priceless, and saved me much time and legwork by allowing me to build on what she has already learned about soy over the years in dealing with the allergy.

I also want to thank all who had a hand in the the book and cover design; I especially want to thank my wonderful daughter, Anahlisha, for her design and illustration work for the cover. She is a fantastic artist and a great collaborator.

It would be impossible to cite in the text all the authorities and sources consulted for this project. The material would be an encyclopedic reference in its own right. I have attempted to be as diligent and thorough as possible during the information gathering process and follow-up fact checking. I have included what I hope is a useful and educational bibliographic and online reference list to get you started; doubtless you will discover many others. This list contains the bulk of my own forays and reading in my personal search to learn about soy and soy allergens. Feel free to write to me with suggestions of what to include in future editions and improvements to make to the guide. If you do, and I use it, I will make sure that you get an acknowledgment for your contribution. I want the guides to be for you, and what can help you cope with an allergy.

I want to thank all who were involved with the copy-editing, proofreading and fact checking. It wouldn't be what it is without your help and considerate input through the whole project: my wife, who was there every step of the way, reading, suggesting, cajoling, questioning, double-checking everything; my daughter, Anahlisha, who has a knack for effectively organizing visual and textual information. Without your help it wouldn't have seen the light of day.

I also want to acknowledge all of the companies and food producers who are becoming more responsive to the needs of a larger cross section of their customer base. During research I was pleasantly surprised by the number of positive changes I've noted toward making products more allergy friendly, or allergy aware is the term I've chosen for this book. It's a hopeful and wonderful sign. Kudos to you.

I also want to emphasize that the names, logos, brands and trademarks of companies and products used in the text were for reference only, and all marks and names are the sole property of the respective owners. No claim of ownership or association should be construed from such inclusion.

DISCLAIMER

This material was designed to provide helpful and accessible information on the subjects discussed and is presented for educational purposes only.

This book is not meant to be used, nor should it be used to diagnose or treat any medical condition. For diagnosis or treatment of any medical condition, consult your personal physician.

The publisher and the author are not responsible for any specific health or allergy needs that may require medical supervision and are not liable for any damages or negative consequences that may incur from any treatment, action, application or preparation to any person reading or following the information in this book.

References are provided for informational purposes only and don't constitute endorsement of any websites or other sources. Readers should be aware that the websites listed in this book may change.

To reiterate for clear understanding, nothing contained in this guide is offered as the final authority; the author is not a doctor or an allergist. All information is derived from personal experience and additional research into the subject of food allergies. The author and publisher shall have neither liability nor responsibility to any person or entity with respect to any loss or damage caused or alleged to have been caused by the information contained in this book.

If you do not wish to be bound by the above you may return this book to the publisher for a full refund.

AUTHOR'S NOTE

Dear Readers

I want you to know that I have done everything in my power to bring you an excellent product that will add value to your life and provide you the answers you need to help your life flow better. It is important for me to assure you that my work is my own, and everything I do is fully checked and rechecked to assure that it meets the highest standards. I base all of my projects on an honest work ethic and I stand behind them 100%.

In light of that, please know that I don't copy or lift the work of others; I do my own research and generate my own dedicated content. When I research I do it in terms of discovering and affirming the facts I need to present my case, from my unique perspective, with cogency and clarity.

I hate plagiarism, and anyone is free to check the veracity of my work at any time. I expend every effort to edit and check my work thoroughly to make sure that it is ready for the wide world; I want you to be able to interact with the work in a valuing, meaningful way devoid of any extraneous worries. Namely, my greatest reward is knowing that something I've produced has helped by some real measure. I will always do everything I can to give you the Baker's Dozen.

When you purchase any of my books or other information products, you can rest assured that you're gaining a useful asset that is the best that I can offer.

I want to thank you for choosing my work to guide you in your quest for answers. I hope I have provided a basis for true results. I'll continue to do my utmost to not let you down. If you would like to provide feedback about your reading experience, I welcome your contact for meaningful and reasonable discussion. Be on the lookout for future volumes in the Food Allergy Guide Series.

Thank you

Bill Bowling
January 10, 2014

CONTENTS

INTRODUCTION

SOY, SOJA, SOYA, SHOYU, TOFU, EDEMAME, by many names...

The indefatigable soybean, Glycine Max if you want to get scientifically fancy about it: Soy has literally taken over our food supply. Soy is in everything—might as well be.

Soy does seem to be everywhere, either as filler, by product or first ingredient. Almost any food product you pick up in the grocery store has a soy derivative in it. Well, you ask, what's wrong with that? It's great filler, it stretches our food supply, it's basically good for you, and it is so plentiful it helps to lower overall food costs. The answer is that there isn't much negative to say about soy according to large numbers who rely on soy daily to meet their dietary needs; well, there is some debate and a few real concerns about the overall effects of soy, but more about that later. The fact is that soy has been a staple in our diets for a few generations.

Soy IS mostly good, and it can be made to look and taste like many other foods. It is basically healthy and it has added greatly to our society as a food product. That's all wonderful; long live the SOYBEAN, right?

Mostly right—unless you've developed a dangerous allergy to it. Then what? If soy is in so many things, what are people with a potentially life-threatening allergy to this miracle legume going to do? How are they going to find wholesome and varied foods to eat that won't potentially kill them? We all got to eat, yes? Yes, we do, and it is possible to do so without soy.

That is what this entry in the Food Allergy Series will address. Soy is one of the eight top food allergens along with wheat, milk, eggs, fish, shellfish, peanuts, and tree (or true) nuts. There are many, many others, interestingly enough—yeast, sulfites, sesame seeds, lupine, celery, and surprising as it may seem, the list could go on and on. I initially came up with the analogy that our food is somehow turning against us, but after some serious reflecting on it, I decided that was wrong thinking; now, I more so think that we are tinkering too much with our food supply, and that is more likely the main causal factor in the increasing number of people with food allergies. All of these allergens need in-depth study, but the focus here is on soy. The rest will get needed attention as we go along, and those study projects are presently in development.

Looking at safe foods, and outlining an overall

strategy for eating well in order to avoid the systemic disturbances that ingesting soy can bring about are the primary focus areas of this book. Also, I want to offer some simple guidelines of what to look for when you're shopping so that you buy only soy-free foods that are safe for you to eat. I'm offering this as your soy allergy handbook/field guide so that you can develop your own safe list based on the foods that you prefer and take the guesswork and uncertainty out of your trips to the grocery store.

You will gain the knowledge you need to manage your food allergy with full confidence. It is always about the educational process. Once you have the education, you have the means to dispel all of that swirling stuff that impedes your progress—stuff like fear, anxiety, frustration.

I'll talk about the history of soy, the presence of soy in our food supply, how to read labels; I'll discuss the debate about soy, and genetic modification, but overall it's about your allergy and how to cope with it, how to deal with it.

I became interested in Food Allergies in general, and got started on my path of tracing soy food products for a personal reason after my wife developed a terrible allergy to soy, and it was stressful simply researching to find out exactly what she could safely eat without fear of going into anaphylactic shock from eating something she loved. Life before the allergy was definitely much simpler; if she wanted a sandwich, she made a sandwich, no problem, no worries. Post allergy, not so simple; that sandwich could be a serious threat. That sandwich could have soy in it —the bread, even the meat could have soy in it. Nothing like playing soy roulette.

Prior to the sudden onset of her allergy to soy, we ate soy products without a thought or a care; we looked at labels to check other nutritional values, but we didn't have any reason to search for soy. All of that changed with the miso soup affair. That's what I call it; it was the miso soup that appeared to have been the catalyst that triggered her immune system to say, "Hell, no, miso, no more soy for you, dear." She really did have an affair with miso—she was eating several bowls a week. It can't be declared absolutely that the miso soup initiated that tipping point, but, even at this time, it seems to be connected.

#

For full revelation, at the time of onset of the soy allergy, my wife was dealing with another health issue that caused her immune system to to be low, and according to research this is a perfect opportunity for other problems to creep in unannounced and wreak additional havoc on the system. In terms of food allergy, the food you've been consuming the most of—remember the miso soup—at the time the allergy starts is what your immune system flags as the allergen.

The interesting thing about soy allergy is that it can start suddenly without any prior indicators. Something alerts those antibodies in the immune system of the individual that then start reading soy as an enemy and fight against it, creating some really scary effects. One line of thought suggests that soy allergy is rare and manageable. It is manageable of course, but no one wants to go through even the minor side effects that ingesting an allergen can cause. So, respectfully, it may not be wise to underrate the experiences of the sufferers. I've seen my wife brought to tears from the itching alone because she ate something that had a hidden soy product.

After confirmation of the allergy, there was a major whirlwind of adjustment activity in our household. We knew zip about soy, and suffice to say it was a very steep learning curve. She was having a hard time figuring out what she could eat, and when she started her research in the attempt to educate herself, the extent of soy in our food came as major shock and surprise. There were more unknowns than knowns.

There were a couple of instances that illustrate this early lack of full knowledge base very well. A short time after that initial outbreak someone offered her a piece of gum, and she accepted it. As a result she had a major flare-up that brought about a scary few days. This happened because she had no idea that chewing gum contains soy. Since then, she has managed to find only one flavor of one particular brand that doesn't contain it. Yes, soy is in chewing gum.

Another early instance, post allergy—she had some information by this time—we were at a party, an outdoor barbeque, picnic with friends, and there was a number of great food dishes, but after checking the ingredients, she was able to eat only a couple of items from the array: Another lesson on the extent of soy.

Early on in the process, she was eating salads with no dressing because it was the safest path to follow. But as time went on she acquired the knowledge she needed to feel comfortable going out to eat, attending functions with family and friends, and preparing food for herself at home. Initially though it was a very serious, unbalanced, disruptive, fearful, uncomfortable, challenging, compromising, and dangerous position to be in; I know that's stacking a lot of adjectives, but I want to paint a clear emotional picture. It required total commitment and change: Change in approach to food; change in diet habits; change in the method and manner of shopping; change in awareness toward a basic function. There was no more taking food for granted. The mandate became to know, always know what you're putting into your body because if you don't it just might kill you.

#

Jump forward to the present, and she has done a great deal to conquer the allergy, and advocate for other sufferers.

This book is the result of that living research into a food allergy and how it can change your life. I'm starting with soy because it is the one that hit close to home, but the others will receive their just due in order to help as many people as possible get a handle on an expanding food problem. Hopefully the information collected here will provide a more accessible package than the mountain of oftentimes conflicting data and statistics out there in cyber land and elsewhere.

As I alluded to earlier, the companion volumes covering the other seven allergens as well as the four or so ones not recognized by the United States but listed in other parts of the world are in development and will be out as soon as I can polish them and get them market ready. You are holding Volume One, and Volume Two focusing on peanuts, another strange and 'nutty' legume, will follow in quick succession.

It's fascinating and concerning that the number of people affected by food allergy is increasing the world over. That definitely bears ongoing, deep study and overdue consideration. We don't know what causes food allergies, but we know something is going on that doesn't bode well for our nutrition and health; we know that food sensitivities and allergies seem to be increasing only in the developed world; we know that there is something happening to our food supply that needs our ongoing assessment.

We can talk about the Hygiene Factor, (the Hygiene Factor poses simply that we are too clean, and as a result of that hyper-cleanliness, our systems are too rarefied, as good a word as any), GMO's and other bugs in our collective reaping of food. Those are all interesting and definitely worth our notice and activism. There's more to come later regarding all of that, but right now, let's learn about soybeans so you get a firmer handle on the allergen. You can eat safely and well without soy! Welcome to the SOY FREE world.

CHAPTER ONE: HISTORY OF SOY

The soybean is native to Asia, and its cultivation can be traced back thousands of years. The Chinese appear to have been the first to farm soy, and to discover many uses for it. Although no exact date can be determined to mark the entry of soy into the culture, a tentative time line can be established starting at around 3,000 years. Though, according to a Chinese legend, (most likely a tall tale invented and interjected into the culture by historians from a later dynasty), the Emperor Shennong, a mythic figure dating back to about 5,000 years ago, declared five grains as sacred food: Soybeans, (we know that soybean isn't a grain, but we quibble), rice, wheat, barley and millet. He has been worshiped as a venerated figure, and his presence is still seen in festivals and such; a rough translation of his name is 'Divine Farmer'. Invented myth or not, the story of

Shennong points out the importance of the soybean, and the high standing the soybean has enjoyed in Chinese culture throughout its history.

#

History is filled to the Grand Bazaar Basket brim with the 'sacred' soybean. It did take a little time making its way out of the orient. But it finally did, in a snail's pace across Asia, middle Asia, the islands, and finally on into Europe and the new colonies that eventually became the United States of America.

In Asia there was a gradual development of soy based foods such as Tofu, and Soy Sauce. It would be a fascinating fact to know just how much soy sauce has been consumed over the millennia since its invention. In ancient times, soy was processed through fermentation and drying, with salt serving as the primary agent. Tofu is made using a simple combination of water, salts, (sometimes acids and enzymes), and soybean paste. Soy Sauce is made by steeping a mixture of boiled soybeans, wheat grain, and yeast mold in a brine of water and salt. Coincidentally, there are some findings to suggest that it is the fermented soy products that are most healthy for all of us. While tofu is not technically a fermented product, there are some fermented tofu varieties: There are basic pinyin, and stinky pinyin, made with a fish brine. Soy sauce certainly is a fermented product.

When we start looking at the history of soy we see the names of some very famous people pop up in relationship to it, prominent people of their respective times whose stories serve to illustrate how the soybean was spread and how it finally made its way to the New World, and how it became such an expansive, pervasive crop. George Washington Carver's name comes up in connection to soy, but that connection is most likely overblown. Benjamin Franklin's name appears in historical references to soy as being the first to introduce soybeans to the new world, but his involvement of sending back some seeds to a friend in Philadelphia from France while he was overseas on a trip in 1770 marks a later time, and does not represent the first introduction of soybeans to America as is sometimes cited in other sources. That distinction probably belongs to Samuel Bowen, who brought seeds back from China in 1765 and later planted them on his land in the Georgia Colony. But I don't want to get ahead of myself. I'll relate more about George Washington Carver, and Henry Ford in a little bit; yes, even Henry Ford had a very interesting connection to soy. We'll talk about it. But first, let's check out Europe.

Soybeans became increasingly present in Europe and other parts of the world at the beginning of the 19th century; prior to that soy remained largely an Asian crop. According to records, missionaries to China sent back seeds to France as early as 1739; that is one of the earliest mentions of soy in Europe. For a long time China remained the largest percentage producer of the soybean supply. At the present time the United States is the major supplier while China is the largest customer.

Soy was very slow to catch on as a food product, and was for the longest time viewed only as compost or as food for cattle. Through all of the testing and trials over the years from the last half of the 19th century and the first quarter of the 20th century, the soybean as food for people was met with mixed reviews, most of them negative.

Let's catch up with George Washington Carver and Henry Ford; George Washington Carver is often associated with the development of soy in America, but his primary work was concentrated in peanuts, (even his connection to peanuts isn't as extensive as we sometimes tend to think), and other than writing a couple of research reports on 'the bean', he wasn't actively connected to the advancement of soybeans. Henry Ford, on the other hand, interestingly enough, had a research facility where he put his bevy of scientists to work on discovering as many uses as possible for soybeans with the result being a soy plastic that was subsequently used on gearshift knobs, pedals, switches, what have you, even to the actual body of his famous automobiles. Suffice to say, Henry Ford used a lot of soybeans. Who knew? Henry Ford and his soy cars.

Soy gained major ground in the 1940's as a foodstuff, and that growth continued during the sixties and seventies. But it was in the nineties at the tail end of the 20th century that soy found its mark. During this new era of the natural food renaissance, soy was magically rediscovered, and became a star; soy continues in the limelight today. Soybean allergy was first reported in 1934; it was in the 1980's that soy began to be labeled as one of the top eight food allergens. Prior to that it was recognized, but it was further down on the list, and not considered a major problem.

One soy product that has seen the greatest develoment over the last few decades is soy milk. Soy milk has been subject to an assertive marketing effort. Introduced in 1978 to the U.S., soy milk saw a major upswing in the 1990s and continues today. SILK has become the premier brand of soy milk. SILK products first appeared in stores in the last few years of the twentieth century, and has grown by leaps and bounds thanks to the efforts of natural food proponents. SILK products use only non-GMO, organically grown soybeans. However, soy milk was known and produced in China for millenia. Soy milk was first mentioned in a book entitled Lunheng by Wang Chong. Yes, it does sound like an album by a funky band.

Soy milk is made by grinding the whole bean in water, and is composed of both the oil and the protein; it practically equals cow milk in protein content. Needless to say, it is literally poison to a soy allergy sufferer. It is covered here to provide as full a profile of the bean as possible, and to show it's strident march through history and geography as a preferred foodstuff.

At this point in history the development of the soybean continues unabated and shows no sign of letting up. Soybean allergy and other food allergies are increasing yearly as well, especially among children, and show no sign of letting up. Hopefully, solid research into what is happening in our food supply will continue alongside all the disruptions. At some point we will have to actually stop, really stop, and take full measure of what we're putting into our bodies that passes as safe nourishment and make some real changes.

The verdict is still out on the ultimate value of the soybean, and meanwhile the tinkering and manipulating will continue, we can assume, and we can only wait and guess the outcomes. Hopefully we aren't creating a monster bean.

The rest of this book will be devoted to working out how to manage your soy allergy, and provide a guide that you can use in the real world to help you make good food choices minus the soybean.

CHAPTER TWO
SOY AND OUR
FOOD SUPPLY

SOY AS FOOD:

Here's an interesting note to start out with: Raw soybeans are toxic to all animals with a single stomach; that includes humans, and indeed most other animals; however, if you are a ruminant—if you have a four chambered stomach—like cattle, you get a pass.

What is soy? Soy is a legume—a bean—sharing a many branching family tree with all other beans or legumes from peanuts to pintos, lentils to limas. The indications are that if you are allergic to one legume, you might be allergic or might eventually become allergic to others in the family. It's an expansive family with a long history of cultivation and use as food; also as important commodities going far back in the cultural history of all peoples of the world.

#

In terms of nutritional value, soybeans are low in cholesterol, high in protein, and they're also a great source of vitamin C, calcium and iron. The soybean is used as a meat substitute; it is used as a milk substitute; it is used as an oil; it is used in infant formula. We could go on and on: Soy is that versatile.

The soybean does have almost inexhaustible uses as filler or as product derived directly or indirectly from the bean. A perhaps surprising thing to discover is that the soybean itself is not a major element in most of our diets, but the wide variety of products rendered from it are.

The two main derivatives from the bean are oil and protein; soy proteins are the primary source of an allergy to soy. Soy oil and oil derivatives don't appear to be as allergenic; the FDA exempts manufacturers from labeling requirements related to soy oil, and you will see soy oil often listed as simply vegetable oil. I'll expand on all of this in later chapters along with what to look for when reading labels so that you can shop safely and confidently.

The seeming simplicity of that revelation would be great for the soy allergy sufferer if that was the extent of it, but it isn't; as we are about to learn there is a very long grocery anti-list of products that have some element of soy in them.

THE EVOLUTION OF SOY:

The ancients used only the bean and what they could render directly from it as food. Otherwise the soybean plant was used as forage or for soil enrichment. The two ancient methods of processing, fermenting and drying, are still used today. As indicated earlier, it is fermented soy products that appear to be the most healthy to consume, and that provide the most nutrients. Perhaps they knew something we don't know or have forgotten. These processes brought us such things as soy sauce, tofu, (only some varieties are fermented), and natto.

The soybean has come a long way in its trek through time to become the supreme rock star of the legume set; as the lead singer of a band called The Lowly Beans, soy has branched off into many different genres. The premier distinction of the soybean is that it is the first mutant; it was the first to be manipulated so that it can withstand the monsoon of pesticides that is showered down on it to keep it weed-free. GMO's, (Genetically Modified Organisms), are a subject that will be covered in some depth in another chapter, but the soybean plant was the first living organism to undergo such modification.

Over time it was discovered that soy protein and soy oil could be manipulated in the same way as animal proteins, and so sprang from soy a seemingly endless variety of chemical products and derivatives that are used in, well, practically everything: pharmaceuticals, foodstuffs, cleaning fluids, disinfectants, cosmetics, toiletries, infant formula, plastics, clothing, and as what is called 'feedstock' in many, many industrial processes; the term feedstock in this case refers to a primary building block in the production of something else. We can give credit to Henry Ford and his research scientists for bequeathing to us the blueprint for the industrialization of soy.

Since its migration out of China, soy has been welcomed and embraced by the whole world, and championed as a wonder food by consumers, special interest groups, commercial growers, producers and distributors alike. It has definitely gone way past the lowly subsistence crop that we imagine it to have been for Chinese farmers as it provided food for both livestock and humans. They grew, harvested, and preserved the bean as best they knew how. But now? Now the soybean is a major commodity; the bean itself and its derivatives generate billions of dollars a year in trade and revenue.

Add to the ancient methods of fermenting, and drying: boiling, reducing, compounding, filtering, separating, extracting, crystallizing, synthesizing, hydrolyzing, isolating, oxidizing, other hocus-pocus tricks of chemistry, and you get an idea of how far soy has come.

Factions that have some form of interest in soy will talk about moderation, but there's a problem; with soy there isn't a point of moderation. At the risk of overemphasizing, we're inundated with soy from every possible direction: we're eating soy in everything, we're wearing soy, we're cleaning with soy, and if you have an allergy, you can't work from moderation standards, you have to work from elimination standards, and if you are allergic, only you know how hard that is, and only you know how silly, inadequate and unreachable some arbitrary condition of use is.

The culture, and here we're talking about global culture, appears to have fully embraced soy, and elevated soy above wheat as the staple we can't do without. The positive notion for the soy allergy sufferer to keep in mind is that there are many alternatives, and soy isn't irreplaceable. You can do without soy. There are even viable alternatives for protein replacement other than soy for vegans and vegetarians; that is, though, a whole other book, and another avenue to explore.

CHAPTER THREE
I'M ALLERGIC TO SOY—WHAT NOW?

CARDINAL RULES FOR DEALING WITH A FOOD ALLERGY:

Let's start this chapter by establishing some important guidelines. I've presented them here as cardinal rules, and that is exactly what they are. You have a food allergy, and that means making some important adjustments in the way you view food, the way you cook food, and the way you interact in social circles that may not be as aware as you now are of the dangers that the target foods pose for you. It ultimately means a whole change in lifestyle. You can't go to a party or an event, or out to a restaurant and eat or order anything that seems appealing. You can't simply accept food that is offered with a gracious thank you; you have to ask, you have to find out what is in it before you eat it. You have to be conscious of every bite so that you stay safe and nourished at the same time. Below are those cardinal rules that you must use as your guide for your whole life:

1. **READ THE INGREDIENT LABELS**
2. **IF IN DOUBT, AVOID IT**
3. **EDUCATE YOURSELF**
4. **BE PROACTIVE; ASK QUESTIONS**
5. **CONTACT THE MANUFACTURERS**

WHAT ARE THE SYMPTOMS?

There is a wide range of symptoms associated with soy allergy:

- Skin breakouts and rashes similar in appearance to eczema
- Swelling of the mouth, throat and lips
- Rhinitis or nasal congestion
- Asthma like symptoms
- Constriction of the airway
- Canker sores and fever blisters
- Colitis, gastrointestinal upset, and diarrhea
- Conjunctivitis (pink eye), not the contagious viral or bacterial variety.
- Feeling weak and extremely fatigued
- Nausea and vomiting

- Itching
- Low blood pressure
- Hay fever
- Hives
- Anaphylactic shock—which is a potentially life-threatening situation

WHAT IS ANAPHYLAXIS?

Anaphylaxis is an extreme reaction to an allergen that can bring about respiratory distress to the point of death in the absence of effective countermeasures.

Anaphylaxis is a dire emergency and requires immediate action. Anyone with a serious allergy to any food product should get, and keep with them at all times, a supply of epinephrine, which is administered by injection through commercially prepared self-injectable devices that are easily acquired with a prescription from a healthcare provider and safely carried in a pocket or bag. There are a few brand names available, and they are all pretty much equal in efficacy, being not much more than a pre-measured, ready dose of adrenaline—Adrenaclick, Auvi-Q, Epipen, and Ject.

Another danger with anaphylaxis is that the symptoms can go away and then return with major consequences several hours later. It can take as little as a few minutes after ingestion for an onset, but it can also be delayed by a few hours. That is why it is very important to always be prepared. There isn't a clear understanding why this happens, but in any situation of compromise continual monitoring is imperative so that there aren't any surprises hours or even as many as two days later.

The cautionary note here is that you shouldn't allow yourself to be lulled into a false sense of security where a catastrophic medical event could be lurking just around the corner. Individuals react differently with exposure to an allergen.

SYMPTOMS OF ANAPHYLAXIS

Anaphylactic shock can involve many body systems:

- **On the skin:** Skin reactions in the form of itching, flushing, development of hives, or swelling, especially of the face, lips, and eyes.

- **In the eyes:** In addition to itching and swelling you will see copious production of tears and redness.

- **Around the nose and mouth:** You will see sneezing, runny nose, nasal congestion, swelling of the tongue. Some people also report a metallic taste.

- **Respiratory system, difficulty breathing:** There will be interference with breathing, repeated coughing, tightness in the chest, wheezing or other breathing problems, increased mucus production, swollen or itchy throat, hoarseness, change in voice, or a choking sensation. These symptoms and the following symptoms are the most severe and present the most danger. Anything that interferes with breathing or circulation requires emergency treatment.

- **Circulatory system, blood pressure drop:** Dizziness, weakness, fainting, rapid, slow, or irregular heart rate and a drop in blood pressure are symptoms that should be addressed as soon as possible after their onset.

- **The digestive system:** Nausea, vomiting, abdominal cramps, and diarrhea.

- **Nervous system:** During Anaphylaxis the person may develop anxiety, confusion, or a sense of impending doom.

As you can see here, the allergy can affect the whole body: Skin, eyes, nose, mouth, respiratory, circulatory, digestive and nervous systems. The main action in a case of suspected anaphylaxis is to get the allergy sufferer to emergency care as quickly as possible.

DIFFERENCE BETWEEN ALLERGY AND INTOLERANCE

Sometimes an intolerance to a certain food is lumped together with an allergy. There is a distinct difference that is important to point out. A preface to that is someone with a sensitivity to a food can develop a full-blown allergy. It is important also in both cases to avoid the food so that you don't have an outbreak. Okay, what is the difference? **An intolerance or sensitivity involves only the gastric, digestive system**. An allergy on the other hand involves the immune system, and is a potentially more dangerous involvement.

SYMPTOMS OF INTOLERANCE

Symptoms can show up immediately after ingestion or can show up days later. If you know that you have a sensitivity, avoiding soy foods is your safest course of action. The symptoms of soy intolerance and allergy can overlap and an occurrence is an emergency if—there is difficulty breathing, extreme swelling of lips, face, and throat; or there is itchy skin, rash or unconsciousness. These emergencies can occur even with a history of mild involvement.

Other symptoms are gastric in nature: gas,

heartburn, bloating, persistent nausea, vomiting, along with uncomfortable sensations in the chest and throat. Migraine headaches are common as are instability, mood and behavioral changes.

44

CHAPTER FOUR
INFANT AND CHILDHOOD ALLERGY

Some data suggest that children will outgrow their food allergy by the age of ten. However, the other side of that assertion is the determination that if a child has an allergy, that child will continue to be sensitive to the target food for the rest of their lives. As well, an allergy can disappear or abate and reappear at a later time dependent on exposure to and ingestion of the target allergen. The special importance of this information for the future, in particular, is that since an ingredient has been determined to be a problem, the allergy sufferer knows to be cautious when coming in contact with suspect products.

Whatever the case, each person's allergy is a phenomenal manifestation with the same etiology yet affects each individual system in a unique way. Relative to soy, some will be able to tolerate the oil derivatives, but others will need to totally eliminate all products that are manufactured with soybeans from their diet. Manufacturers can't offer a full guarantee that all protein elements are extracted during the processing of the beans and the manufacturing of the oil; in that sense alone, your thinking should be that the allergen is present unless it is proven otherwise. That is your safest course.

Childhood allergies need to be handled a little differently than adults: First of all, children need help to manage their allergy, and second, their social circles are a bit different and there are times during their day when they are away from their parents and primary caretakers. It is very important for parents to educate others regarding their child's needs. It is also very important for parents to educate their child about allergens and how to avoid exposure; make sure your child understands that he or she shouldn't accept free food, or exchange food with friends due to the possibility of accidentally ingesting the allergen. Warn your child to be extra careful in school situations such as classroom parties, and around any outside food such as fund-raising bake sales and such. Yes, Girl Scout cookies have soy.

#

Infants are in yet another category altogether in that their progress and situation will be looked after cooperatively with parent and pediatrician. We'll return to childhood allergies later, but first let's look at the special situation surrounding babies and infant formula.

INFANTS AND SOY FORMULA

A baby's system is delicate; the potential issue with soy formula is the harsh quality of the soy protein. Soy is proven to be highly allergenic. It is very important for parents to communicate with the family physician and the infant's pediatrician regarding any observed extreme reactions to soy formula. Babies will show sensitivity to soy by excessive spitting up, or will display abdominal pain after eating by crying inconsolably, flailing arms and rolling into a fetal position. If your baby is exhibiting sensitivity, your doctor needs to know as soon as possible to prescribe an alternative that will keep your little one safe and nourished. There are a number of alternatives, and I want to outline and talk about each from the most desired to the least:

BREAST MILK

The optimal choice in any circumstance would be what is the most natural. In this case that is the natural bond between mom and baby through breast feeding. Of course, there isn't any negative association to be inferred in relation to a mother not being able to breast feed. For many reasons, some mothers can't. It's merely to indicate that breast milk is the best for baby. Actually, infant formulas are created to approximate what the baby gets from mother's own milk, but none have been able to reproduce its nutritional perfection. Breast milk is the perfect nutritional match for baby. This wonder food is made up of a primo blend of fats, cholesterol, carbohydrates, proteins, vitamins, minerals, and other constituents that are still being studied. The very interesting thing about breast milk is that its composition changes as the baby grows and develops so that solid foods can be gradually introduced till the child is fully weaned off the milk.

#

As stated, some mothers don't have the means to breast feed; some simply choose not to for personal and religious reasons. In those cases, the alternative is formula, but in the case of a food allergy, mom and doctor will need to team up in order to determine the best product for baby's nutrition. Rest assured with the knowledge that your infant will be adequately nourished with formula, but know also that it is only a close approximation to breast milk; it ain't what mama makes. I couldn't resist, folks, I couldn't resist. For another piece of important information, it has also been shown that if an infant shows extreme sensitivity to soy based formula, he or she may show an intolerance to cow milk based formula as well. If you and your doctor work in concert for the benefit of your baby, everything should be fine, with breast feeding or without.

AMINO ACID BASED FORMULA

If you've tried other formulas and it's been determined that your baby is adversely reacting to both milk and soy-based formulas, your pediatrician can prescribe a third option, which is an amino acid formula. NEOCATE, ELECARE, and NUTRAMIGEN AA are common brands of amino acid-based formulas. Amino acid formulas are different in the way that protein is used. Amino acids are the most simple forms of protein, and are not as harsh for baby's system.

GOAT MILK

Another viable alternative is goat milk. Goat milk has many benefits for those children who can't tolerate cow milk. There are also laboratory based findings that rank goat milk over cow milk because of its general make up: Goat milk has less of the protein Alpha s1, which subsequently makes it less of an allergen than cow milk. Goat milk has been found to be a better match for the human system, is easier to digest because of the lower lactose content, and goat milk doesn't separate like cow milk, so it doesn't need to go through the artificial homogenization process; it is naturally homogenized. Homogenization is the process where the fat globules are forced through a filter to make them smaller, causing the milk product to stay together and not separate.

HOMEMADE BABY FORMULA

You can make your own, but before considering it, you will need to fully educate yourself, and know exactly, scientifically what you need to put together so that you don't rob your baby of fundamental nutritional values and interfere with his proper development. In other words, if you don't know what you are doing you can harm your baby by feeding her a homemade concoction that isn't adequate for her needs. Breast milk is the highest benchmark, and that is always what we strive for, but barring that, prepared infant formulas are scientifically created to assure that the product is as close a facsimile of the real thing as possible. With homemade formula, you can achieve the same thing, but you will have to do some rather extensive research—this can't be stressed too much—to find the correct recipe with the right combination of ingredients so that your baby is adequately nourished. It isn't something to debate, create conflict around, or be defensive about; if you decide that this is the direction you need to go in, arm yourself with the right skills and concern for the benefit of your baby.

Fact is, there are some concerns about the overall safety of established formulas, but that debate is ongoing with no clear answers yet. One thing is certain: toxic additives, non-nutrients, anti-nutrients are finding their way into all of our foodstuffs; we do need to start questioning more and more why they are there, and infant formulas are no exception, high levels of melamine, and other nasty things. The point being that one of the major pros of making your own formula is that you will be more in control of what you're feeding your baby. The other major point is that sense of independence is laudable but it needs to be balanced by full commitment on your part so that your baby is safe and nourished. Your baby's health always comes first, over any belief, and over any polarizing political posturing. We're talking here about a potential medical issue that could go beyond sensitivity and intolerance to more systemic problems if not handled right from the beginning. The first few months of your baby's life are very important in terms of fundamental development. Enough said; I'll move on.

The problem with making your own formula is that there are many recipes floating around; you can find many on the internet, through word of mouth from friends, and other sources. Those could be good or they could be lacking in some important thing. Don't simply whip up the first thing you come upon without checking and comparing as well as considering the source. Not all recipes are created equal. The recommended primary ingredient is goat milk, and from there you can go in a few directions with the other ingredients for building a viable formula. I'm not going to provide a ready-to-make formula recipe here. This is just too important to be casual about. Another valuable ingredient is coconut oil for the reason that it contains a high level of lauric acid, which is a natural constituent of breast milk.

If you've decided that you want to go in this direction, the first step is to talk with your child's doctor so that he or she is on the same page with you; perhaps your doctor can even help you develop a recipe. Second you'll need to be diligent with measuring and storage; the measuring has to be precise from batch to batch, and the recommendation is to buy measuring tools that you can dedicate solely to creating your formula. The other part is you'll only want to make up small batches at a time, no more than enough for two days feedings.

#

At the time of writing there isn't consensus on the number of people, adults and children, affected by soy, either from full-blown allergy or intolerance, but that number is surprisingly high. The number of babies adversely affected by soy infant formulas are high as well. Other sources say that if a baby shows sensitivity to milk, he will also show sensitivity to soy; that figure can be as high as 50%. Soy allergy is at roughly 4% for infants, or 4 out of 100.

One of the main problems with soy formula is its prevalence; it is the automatic choice, the prescribed option for families all over the world. Poverty plays a role in that dynamic because soy is a cheap alternative and can be stretched to serve the masses. There isn't, however, any proven relationship between the widespread use of soy, and the rising incidence of reported allergy. You, the parent, are the best advocate for your child. You're there at the beginning, and the best measure is to monitor constantly to make sure your infant is adjusting to his formula. If you see something wrong, make sure your baby's doctor works with you to make needed changes.

Here's a quick run-through of things to look out for with regard to your baby's adjustment to his source of nourishment:

- **Colic**—You hear talk of colicky babies, and it's important to have a clear idea of what colic is. There are a lot of folksy anecdotes related to colic, and everybody knows the word, but not always what it means. First of all colic is your baby's way of trying to communicate with you; your baby can't tell you she is uncomfortable, or hurting, but nature provides ways for babies to signal when something isn't right: irritability, inconsolable crying, fussiness, unusual spitting up, and the most important thing about this is that if it is a problem with the formula, these behaviors will get worse after eating. So colic then is a blanket word we use to describe a set of behaviors that our baby uses to tell us she or he is in distress, and that distress usually stems from an abdominal or a gastric problem.

- **Gas**—Baby gas goes along with colic. Gas can cause your baby serious pain. Some gas, as affirmed by doctors, is normal, but there is a point where it may signal a larger problem: if the gas is unusual in duration; if your baby's stomach is very distended; and if your baby is displaying extreme, ongoing discomfort, it could indicate an allergen as the cause. Also, if your baby is having trouble passing gas, you need to talk with your doctor.

- **Diarrhea**—If your baby is allergic to either soy or milk, his or her delicate gastric system will be in disarray. Diarrhea can indicate a problem with diet. The important thing to keep in mind is that babies poop a lot anyway, and that poop can be messy. Anyone who has ever changed a diaper knows that. For that reason, it is hard to tell what constitutes diarrhea. Here's the key: It only becomes problematic if you see certain things such as sudden changes in bowel habits, very runny, watery stool, or blood in the stool. If these changes are accompanied by rashes, or swelling around the mouth and face that threatens to cut off air supply, it is an emergency. Diarrhea also rapidly causes dehydration, which in turn creates a different medical problem that needs quick attention.

- **Rash**—Rashes such as hives, eczema, (listed separately), are common with food allergies. A rash is the first readable sign that something might be wrong with your baby's diet, and that changes need to be made. If you note any redness, raised patches, diaper rash or skin changes on other parts of your child's body that seems to get worse, contact your doctor to determine the cause.

- **Eczema**—Eczema is irritated red patches that can cause your baby to have serious discomfort. Another name for eczema is atopic dermatitis. The important thing, in this context, is that eczema can be a symptom of something going wrong in your baby's diet. An allergy to soy formula should be considered in cases of eczema if you are using that formula for your baby's nourishment. Other environmental and topical allergens can trigger dermatitis as well, so it's important to get your doctor's help in determining what the cause might be.

  Our daughter was constantly breaking out with a rash for the first few months of her life, and we tried everything to figure out what was causing it, to no avail. Finally, it was discovered that she was reacting to the little metal snaps on the onesies we were dressing her in. After we changed those out, the rash went away. The point is that a number of things in the environment can bring about a reaction, so it's very important to stay alert to any signals that all is not right with your baby, and keep your doctor informed about any changes, no matter how slight they might seem. It is always best to get an answer for any nagging question you might have, and never be embarrassed to ask.

SOY ALLERGY IN TODDLERS AND CHILDREN

Let's look at soy allergy in young children. This is the age where children will start to be outside your scope as the primary caregiver, and you will want to make sure that everyone involved in your child's day-to-day care knows that he or she has an allergy, and you want to be assured that the knowledge is there, and that all involved in care-taking know what to do in case of a problem.

Education is the key at this age. Older children are going to spend time in daycare or school, and anything can happen. Kids love to share food, trade food, accept food that others may not want, and if there isn't a way to determine what's in it, the end result could be a serious medical situation. This is what you don't want. Everyone involved with care needs to have full information to keep your baby safe while he is outside the range of your direct care. You, as the parent or primary caregiver, need to be a firm and willing advocate and make sure that nothing is done without your input or permission. Here are some general guidelines:

- Prepare your child's food at home and send with her. This isn't always possible, but it can take away a lot of worry.

- Provide instructions to school officials and cafeteria staff at school so they're aware of your child's special diet requirements.

- Make it clear that your child shouldn't receive any food if it is not clearly known what is in it.

- Educate your child about the allergen, make sure he or she understands not to take food from anyone.

- Make sure your child has access to antihistamine and an adrenaline injector should the need arise.

- You could have your child wear an alert bracelet and also carry a card.

- Educate others about the allergen and what they need to look out for.

Some sources say that children will outgrow their allergies by age five; others say by the age ten. Conflicting information abounds regarding childhood allergies, that leaves parents uncertain about a direction to go in for reliable answers and wondering how to look at the long term prospects. The other likelihood is, and it has been stated in other sections, that if a child reacts to a food allergen in childhood, he or she will be sensitive to the allergen throughout life; that is the most likely situation. This is a possibility that definitely needs to be considered. With that knowledge, it is advisable for the allergic child to be cautious in using a product that he's been known to react to negatively in the past. Allergies can also subside and return at a later time; this is something to keep in mind as well.

In the case of soy allergy, children can become allergic to other members of the legume family that includes everything from peanuts to lentils; this entails carefully monitoring the ingestion of these foods, especially peanuts, to make sure there aren't multiple allergens. It is a common pattern that a child who is allergic to soy will be allergic to peanuts.

#

As a general summary for this section, here are some things that are known about childhood allergies:

- Boys react more to food allergens on the whole than girls.
- The economic impact of childhood food allergies is over $25 billion per year.
- Available figures put the drastic jump in

reported food allergies between 1997 and 2007 at 18%. If that figure points to a trend, then from then to the present, that figure would be higher.

- Food allergies among children account for 50%.
- Food allergies in children will invariably involve more than one condition—asthma, and associative allergens, i.e, more than one allergy.

60

CHAPTER FIVE
HOW TO MANAGE
YOUR SOY ALLERGY

If your immune system is low, you are more susceptible to developing an allergy to soy, in particular, because it is in so many products. You can develop an allergy to soy at any age, and it comes about in a lot of cases because there are other attendant problems, (especially metabolic issues), and the body interprets the soy product as an invader and begins to fight it off by releasing antibodies, and this is what brings about the allergic reaction and the barrage of symptoms that can include major skin breakouts such as eczema and hives on through a spectrum to life-threatening respiratory problems.

#

How do you manage your soy allergy once it's determined that you have it? Well, your life will change, and you will have to learn some new habits related to food: You will have to shop differently; you will need to cook differently, and if you eat out or attend functions that are outside you control, you will need to make others aware so that your needs can be attended to. Most restaurants don't see a problem with soy, and most will only have a few menu items that are soy free. You need to learn to speak up and advocate for yourself.

The good news with respect to eating out is that there is expanding awareness, and some restaurants have begun to add a separate list of potential allergens in their menu offerings so that diners can make safe choices based on their needs.

Here's the rest of the bad news first: The bad news is that once you develop the allergy, it won't reverse itself, or go away, and very well can become worse if you continue to ingest soy in any form. There is also, unfortunately, no cure for a food allergy.

There is conflicting information regarding infants and children with soy allergy. A lot of sources indicate that infants and children will grow out of their allergy, but the incidence is relatively low, and even those who do seem to outgrow the allergy to some degree remain sensitive to the target food throughout their lives. There really isn't any definitive study to prove this one way or the other. That's important to reiterate and it's also important to reiterate that adults who have a soy allergy won't see a reversal.

The key to managing a food allergy is avoidance of the offending food; in the case of soy, even though some soy products are touted as less allergenic than others, it's best to be fully safe by avoiding all products that might contain soy in any form.

ALLERGY MANAGEMENT GUIDELINES:

- **EDUCATE YOURSELF:** Do your own research and find out as much as you can about soy allergy: How it is likely to affect you, and what you can do over the long haul to prevent potentially life-threatening situations. The more you learn about soy and what it is, the less likely you are to be surprised. An important fact, for instance is that if you are allergic to soy, you are likely to develop an allergy to other legumes, especially lentils and peanuts. My wife has been able to eat both without any problems. She is very cautious and tests with minute portions before eating a full serving. This is critically important knowledge because it mandates caution about consuming these foods as well. The intention with this book is to give you a solid foundation so that you gain the core knowledge you need to change your eating habits away from grub and go let's say to more conscious involvement, and to make the lifestyle adjustments required for your well-being. I've included a bibliography and other resources to provide a means for you to add to your knowledge base in order to expand your education.

- **ASK QUESTIONS:** It is important to be as proactive as possible especially when you are out and about at restaurants, at special gatherings, at family events where your friends and loved ones may not be as cognizant as you about soy and its effects. You need to ask questions; don't be afraid to ask restaurant staff and management about what is in the food you might order, or how it is prepared. Talk to friends and family members if you will be attending an event outside your home, and make them aware of your needs, and how they can help you with your allergy. Always make sure you know what is in any food that is offered to you so you won't be surprised and end up suffering with a dangerous outbreak, or in the hospital.

- **READ LABELS:** Attempting to provide a list of every food or household item on the average grocery shelf would be almost impossible. Instead of approaching it from the perspective of brand names and specific foodstuffs, concentrate instead on carefully reading labels to determine if what you are planning to buy contains soy. A list of what to look for is provided in a separate chapter. You should not buy a product if a label indicates soy or soy derived products, soy flour, mono-diglycerides, diglycerides or lecithin. There are many more, and they're included in this guide.

- **BUY WHOLE FOODS:** Buy whole foods when you can, especially fresh fruit and vegetables, and cook foods yourself with the least number of additives as possible; in that way you will be assured of getting food that is allergen free, and you can relax in the knowledge that you know where everything came from, and how it was prepared. Seek out any specialty stores that might be in your area, and check out the special sections in your regular grocery store for any organic or allergy aware foods. Research and seek out the brand names of companies that produce allergy aware products. A resource list is included in a separate section of this book to get you started. Arming yourself with knowledge and reference sources takes away the anxiety and the guesswork.

- **AVOID PROCESSED FOODS:** Processed foods include foods that have been fully cooked with extra additives and fillers from the production facility, boxed kits such as cake mixes, dinner mixes, canned foods, among others, and it is a sure bet that the bulk of those processed foods will have soy as one the ingredients, sometimes more than one.

- **CARRY BENADRYL:** BENADRYL, generic, diphenhydramine, is an antihistamine that is useful for treating the symptoms of allergies including itching, sneezing, runny nose, skin breakouts, watery eyes, and sinusitis. BENADRYL is great for alleviating the minor symptoms of an allergic reaction to a soy product, but it won't address other more serious, potentially life-threatening processes related to anaphylactic shock. For those emergency situations you would need other stronger medications.

- **ALWAYS CARRY EPINEPHERINE:** It is important that you are always prepared for an outbreak, and possibly anaphylaxis, so you should get and keep with you a viable shot of epinephrine. Epinephrine is nothing more than adrenaline, but it can be a lifesaver. The only stipulation to getting the loaded injectors is that you need to get a prescription from the doctor. Learn how to use the injectors and be sure that you are ready to take action should the need arise.

You should only use epinephrine in a case of extreme emergency.

- **MAKE THINGS FROM SCRATCH:** It sounds like way too much trouble, but it can be fun and rewarding if you approach it with the right spirit. You get the added bonus of enjoying food that has been prepared to your specifications. You avoid all of the unneeded additives, and assure yourself of other health benefits in the process.

- **CONTACT THE MANUFACTURERS:** If you need more information for your peace of mind, call or email the manufacturer to determine what is in the food you or your loved ones intend to eat.

YOUR DOCTOR'S ROLE IN CONTROLLING FOOD ALLERGY:

At some point in your battle with the dreadful food allergen, your doctor will become involved with both treatment and management. He or she may refer you to an allergist for more specialized input. He or she may want you to get an allergy test done to confirm the allergy, and to determine if more than one allergen may be involved in your outbreaks. Allergy tests are of three types—or two depending on the source—consisting of blood testing, skin testing, or patching, (the patch test is sometimes categorized with skin tests); skin tests are the most commonly used to determine food allergies. The bullet points below give a quick rundown of the tests for clarification:

- Blood Testing: This is called the **ELISA** test, or enzyme-linked immunosorbent assay. The ELISA gauges the level of an antibody known as IgE, (immunoglobulin E) in the blood to determine the presence of certain allergens. This test doesn't yield a high level of accuracy, and is rarely used to determine the presence of food allergens. It is also the most expensive test to perform. A **RAST** or radioallergosorbent test can be used as follow up. A third test that is used is the **immunoCAP** or immunoassay capture test for more definitive findings.

- Skin Tests: The **skin prick test** uses small droplets of known allergen solutions that are introduced to the skin and the skin is then either pricked or scratched to cause the solution to enter the body. If the skin reacts with the production of a wheal, (a raised, circular, red, itchy spot at the point of entry), you have positive confirmation of the allergen. Then there is the **intradermal test**; this test is identical in process to the tuberculin skin test that is requisite for certain jobs. An allergen solution is injected just under the skin, and any results noted. If the wheal is present, the test is positive for the allergen. The intradermal test is prone to yielding false positives, but is the most sensitive of all the tests.

• Patch: The **patch test** is sometimes used for determining food allergy. The allergen solution is introduced to the skin by way of a patch that is left on for up to 72 hours. The test is primarily used to check for topical allergies to plants, plastics, and other materials such as soaps, shampoos, lotions, etc.

ALLERGY THERAPY:

The leading statement for this section is that immunotherapy, known as allergy shots, is not effective for food allergy, and rarely used in that context. Allergy therapy consists of a planned series of shots with increased doses and reduced frequency from twice a month to once a month spread over 5 years as a typical regimen. Your doctor administers the shots in the office, and you will be required to stay for a few minutes each time to make sure you don't have any adverse reactions. The medical purpose with the treatments is to introduce controlled amounts of the allergen into the compromised system over certain prescribed time periods; those procedures cause a tolerance to be built up to the allergen and the allergy will fade. The rather extensive shot therapy doesn't cure your allergy, but it may reduce the number and severity of onsets.

CHAPTER SIX
SOY PRODUCTS
AND SOY DERIVATIVES

The products in this section should be straight forward, and avoiding them should be easy for the soy allergy sufferer, but they too can be missed on occasion if they are blended or not listed properly on food labels. It is still widely believed that soy allergy is not a major problem, only a minor annoyance, but it should be noted that anything that can bring about anaphylaxis is not something to be taken lightly.

SOY DERIVATIVES:

- **SOY FLOUR:** Here is where the allergy sufferer can run into a lot of trouble. Soy flour is a product created by grinding the soybeans to a fine powder. Soy flour is literally used in all kinds of foods from candies, pasta, baked goods, meats and yes, even seafood.

- **SOY NUTS:** Soy nuts are whole soybeans that have been soaked in water and then baked till they are crisp and brown. They are billed as an alternative to peanuts due to their similar taste and consistency. They can be flavored with spices or dipped in chocolate. Look carefully to be sure that there is no mix-up in the process of making a purchase.

- **SOY MILK:** Soy milk is pretty much self-explanatory. Soy milk is created through a process of soaking then pressing or grinding the beans in water. The liquid that comes from this process is the soy milk. Additives are then put into the milk to fortify it, flavor it and thicken it. Soy milk is offered in your dairy aisle with regular milk and alternative dairy products. It should be obvious that if you are allergic to soy you should not use soy milk. Soy milk is marketed as a viable alternative to people who want to change their dietary habits. Sometimes you will see something labeled as a soy drink. None of these products are safe for a person with a soy allergy.

- **SOY SPROUTS:** Soy sprouts are simply the sprouts of soybeans. They are full of vitamin C, but thankfully for the soy allergy sufferer, mung bean sprouts and alfalfa sprouts are also available; however, you have to make sure of what you are buying if you don't sprout your own. This is not an area of great concern in this context. Soy sprouts are highly allergenic, but direct products should be clearly labeled and mix ups should be rare.

- **SOYBEAN CURDS, (TOFU):** Soybean curds or tofu as it is commonly called is made with only water, the soy milk and an agent for causing coagulation such as salts, acids, or enzymes which creates the curds. Tofu is created by pressing the curds into forms so that they bind together.

- **VEGETABLE OIL:** Some vegetable oils are made with soy; it is important in this instance to read labels so you won't be surprised by a hidden soy product. The problem is that the label may say vegetable oil, but will be soybean oil. You can either contact the manufacturer or buy a specific oil such as canola, palm, peanut or corn oil; that would remove the guesswork.

- **LECITHIN:** Lecithin is a fatty acid that is used as an emulsifier, as an agent to keep foods from going stale too soon, and to prevent sticking. Lecithin is mainly a by-product of soybean oil, and is used both in food processing—animal and human—and in medicine. Lecithin isn't as allergenic as other products, but where there is even a slight chance of a reaction, it's best to apply the law of avoidance. Lecithin can also be derived from other vegetable sources.

- **SOY PROTEIN:** Soy protein is the basic derivative of the soybean. It is rendered as a powder that is used for filler or as a primary ingredient in vegetarian food or as a red meat alternative.

- **TEXTURED VEGETABLE PROTEIN (TVP):** Textured Vegetable Protein, or TPV, is a flour product and is what is left over after the oil is extracted. TPV is sold as chunks or flakes. It is used as a meat extender and a meat substitute, having a consistency of ground meat after it is hydrated. TPV is also know as Textured Soy Protein (TSP), **Soy Meat** or **Soya Chunks**. It is a vegetarian staple.

- **TEXTURED SOY PROTEIN (TSP):** Check the entry above; Textured Soy Protein is the same as Textured Vegetable Protein. It is used in vegetarian diets as a meat substitute.

- **HYDROLYZED PLANT PROTEIN:** The hydrolyzing process involves boiling the soybean in Hydrochloric Acid then neutralizing the acid by rinsing it with Sodium Hydroxide. This scary sounding process renders a liquid that contains the separated constituents of the beans in the form of amino acids and glutamic acid, which most people know as Monosodium Glutamate or (MSG). MSG is a famous or infamous flavor enhancer that has received a lot of press over the years. Hydrolyzed proteins and MSG are at the center of long running debates as to their overall safety and value in our food supply. MSG has been removed from scores of foodstuffs.

- **HYDROLYZED SOY PROTEIN (HSP):** Hydrolyzed soy protein is another name for Hydrolyzed Vegetable Protein (HVP) and hydrolyzed plant protein (HPP); see under those entries.

- **HYDROLYZED VEGETABLE PROTEIN (HVP):** Hydrolyzed Soy Protein; see the entries for plant protein.

- **NATURAL & ARTIFICIAL FLAVORINGS:** Often indicates the presence of soy.

- **VEGETABLE GUM:** There are a few gums, which originate from different sources: Seaweed, animal tissue, and various plants, including soy, and you won't know what the source is unless you ask the manufacturer or it is revealed on the label. In most cases it will be shown with the source in parentheses such as **'xanthan gum (soy)'**. The variety of gums to look at are Agar Agar, Cellulose Gum, Xanthan Gum, Guar Gum, Locust Bean Gum, and Pectin. Vegetable gums are used as thickeners. Xanthan Gum is usually an indicator of soy in foods.

- **VEGETABLE STARCH:** Vegetable starch in the label usually points to a hidden source of soy. Many vegetables, fruits and grains contain starch.

- **VITAMIN E:** Vitamin E has a connection to soy because of tocopherol-acetate, which is, more often than not, a soy derivative. Be sure to look on the label carefully for the presence of vitamin E/tocopherol-acetate. Tocopherols can be from other sources such as corn; if there is a question about the source of the vitamin E in a product you intend to purchase because the label isn't clear, ask the manufacturer before you buy it and use it.

SOYBEAN FOOD PRODUCTS:

- **ABURA-AGE:** Abura-Age is fried tofu.

- **ATSU-AGE:** Atsu-age is fried tofu.

- **BAKED GOODS:** There are many reasons why you will find soy in virtually all commercially produced baked goods, (there are a few items mixed in with the mountain of soy-based products that are soy free, but you will have to search hard to find them; that is why specialty stores are your friends). The most looming reason is that soy is cost effective in mass production; it is touted as more healthy for you; and less allergenic—of course, the reference is to wheat and other allergies, not soy; it is believed that it makes baked goods look better, and makes food taste better according to customer feedback. It is soy flour we're talking about here that is the main culprit in baked goods.

- **CANNED GOODS, SOUPS:** Look at canned foods carefully before you buy; a lot do contain soy. If there are any doubts about a product after thoroughly reading the label, avoid it, or contact the manufacturer.

- **CEREALS:** A lot of cereals contain more than one soy derivative; thankfully, there are a lot of choices out there that offer good soy free alternatives. Usually the labels are easy to read and decipher.

- **GAN-MODOKI:** Gan-Modoki is a soy dumpling.

- **GLYCINE MAX:** Glycine Max is the fancy name for the soybean; it's mentioned here because you will sometimes see it listed as an ingredient on the label. You need to know that Glycine Max is soy.

- **INFANT FORMULA:** Phytoestrogens are the main causes of concern regarding the use of soy infant formula. Soy infant formula is manufactured as an alternative for infants who can't tolerate milk-based formula or who can't, for various reasons, breast feed. Phytoestrogens, or plant estrogens, act like estrogen in the body, and can potentially cause an overload, which can then bring about cumulative developmental problems that won't be seen till much later in the child's life.

- **KINAKO, (JAPANESE WORD FOR SOY FLOUR):** These distinctions are important to be aware of so that you have the full knowledge you need to shop wisely.

- **NATTO:** With a smell like pungent cheese, natto is a dish of fermented soybeans; it has a slimy texture and a very strong taste that take some getting used to. By some reckoning, natto has been present in Japan from the ninth century. It is fermented with *Bacillus subbilis,* which is prevalent in the human gut, and is considered beneficial.

- **NIMAME:** Nimame is a dish of stewed soybeans.

- **MISO:** Miso is a fermented blend of barley, rice and soybeans, which merits its inclusion here. Fermentation is achieved with a mixture of salt and a type of fungus called *Koji or Kojikin.*

- **SOY SAUCE:** The soy sauce that we are used to, basic soy sauce, is created with a process of fermentation; boiled soybeans, grain, and *Aspergillus oryzae*, a fungus, are placed in a brine of salt and water and allowed to steep for a period of time. The fluid is pressed out of this mixture, and this constitutes the sauce. Soy sauce was invented in China and is thousands of years old. Other names for soy sauce include: **Shoyu, Toyo, Kekap**.

● **TAMARI:** Tamari is Japanese soy sauce in contrast to the original soy sauce that we are more accustomed to seeing; tamari is made with a greater proportion of soybeans than traditional soy sauce.

● **TEMPEH:** Tempeh was first formulated in Indonesia rather than China or Japan. It is fermented soy cake that usually comes to the marketplace wrapped in banana leaves. Tempeh is unique in that it is a whole soybean product. Similar to tofu, but somewhat different in nutritional value and texture, it is like a very firm patty. Tempeh is used in vegetarian cooking as a meat substitute.

● **VEGETABLE BROTH:** There is a difference between stock and broth: Stock is more hearty, and is used for gravies and sauces, while broth is not so concentrated, and is used for soups, etc. Commercial broths do contain soy products in the form of MSG and hydrolyzed soy protein along with natural, artificial colorings and flavorings. There are some brands that don't have a lot of allergens in them, but you do have to explore and patiently search. A safe and delicious alternative is to make your own.

● **WORCESTERSHIRE SAUCE:** Some brands of Worcestershire sauce may have soy as an ingredient, and soy allergy sufferers need to exercise caution in using it; read labels carefully, and avoid the product if unsure of it or contact the manufacturer.

● **YUBA:** Yuba is called tofu skin, bean curd skin, bean curd sheet, or bean curd robes; its use dates back to the 16th century in China and Japan. Soy milk is boiled and the film that develops on top is lifted off and can be used fresh, half dried or dried.

OTHER SOY DERIVATIVES AND BY-PRODUCTS:

The products in this section are a little harder to detect as being soy. These are important to learn so that you can read labels with full confidence.

● **GUAR GUM:** Guar Gum is a powder rendered from the Guar bean; as a pure product, it has no effect on people with a soy allergy, and is therefore safe to use. But soy proteins are added to the Guar Gum, and in light of that information it should be avoided by the soy allergy sufferer. Contact the manufacturer if you have doubts. The ratio is around 10% protein additives; again, avoidance is the safest course.

- **ZANTHAN OR XANTHAN GUM:** Xanthan Gum or zanthan gum is derived from the bacteria *Xanthomonas Campestrias*, and is used as a thickener and stabilizer. It is used in gluten free cooking and serves to replace the gluten in bread making. The relationship to soy allergy is that the Xanthan Gum can retain some traces of the source of the gum, which can be corn, soy, and others. The best course for a person with a soy allergy is to avoid the food in question or contact the manufacturer to determine the source of the Xanthan Gum.

- **TOCOPHEROL-ACETATE:** Tocopherol was covered in an earlier section, but it deserves a listing under its own moniker; *tocopherol-acetate* is vitamin E or vitamin E acetate.

- **YEAST EXTRACT:** Yeast extract is a form of MSG; there may be some who would debate this direct association, but that is what it is, basically. Yeast extract is produced by breaking down the yeast into its constituent parts, removing the covering from the yeast cell, and harvesting the contents of the yeast cell; that extract is used as a flavor enhancer. It can be found in paste, liquid, and powder form.

- **AUTOLYZED YEAST EXTRACT:** Autolyzed yeast extract is the expanded name of yeast extract denoting the process of separation. As indicated above, yeast cells are broken down, and the cell contents are gleaned minus the cell coverings, which yields a monosodium facsimile; that product is used to enhance the flavor of processed foods. Even though a version of monosodium glutamate is present, it doesn't have to be labeled, which is information that you need to know to make decisions about what to buy and consume. Although not technically a soy product, there are some indications that soy allergy sufferers are also sensitive to MSG, plus MSG should be avoided on basic nutritional principle—don't consume anything that may have more negative effects on your body than positive ones.

- **AKARA:** Akara is an African fried food traditionally made with peas, but has been tampered with and changed over time through different influences to include soy products. It doesn't normally contain soy. If you are going to eat Akara, make sure you are consuming a product that is soy free.

- **OKARA:** Okara is soy pulp; it is what's left over after the production of soy milk and tofu. The bulk of it is fed to livestock. It is mainly used as an additive in vegetarian cuisine. There are three kinds of soy protein fibers: Okara, Soy Bran (ground soybean hulls), and soy protein isolate.

- **ISOLATES:** protein Isolates are in powder form and can come from different sources, soy being the main one; isolates are added to a lot of foods, which range from meat substitutes to muscle building protein powders and shakes. If you're allergic to soy make sure you read labels carefully for any item you're interested in. You are looking for soy protein isolate, isolates, or similar designations on the label in the context of soy allergy.

- **OLEAN:** There is a soybean version of OLEAN/OLESTRA; this now mostly defunct experiment by Proctor and Gamble was not originally a soy product. Olestra is still in a few snack foods, potato chips, etc. This is an easy one to avoid; don't buy products with Olean on basic principle.

- **GUM ARABIC:** Gum Arabic is technically from the Acacia tree, and isn't an allergen, but in connection with soy, if it is included on a label it could indicate the presence of added soy protein.

- **BULKING AGENT:** If listed on the label, it can indicate the presence of soy protein.

- **CAROB:** Carob is derived from a member of the legume family, and isn't soy; it is used as a chocolate substitute, and the soy allergy sufferer should be careful about using it as it could become an associative allergen. Plus: its inclusion will sometimes indicate the presence of added soy protein.

- **EMULSIFIER:** Usually indicates the presence of soy derivatives.

- **PROTEIN EXTENDER:** There are a number of key words that can reveal hidden soy. Protein extender is a key phrase; this usually reveals that a compound is present in order to stretch the yield of a certain product, usually meat.

- **STABLIZER:** Can reveal the presence of hidden soy.

- **STARCH:** A listing of starch on the label can reveal the presence of hidden soy. Many other foodstuffs contain starch and are not soy. Use caution here, and find out for sure what it is, and the source of it. The manufacturers can tell you.

- **THICKENER:** Can reveal the presence of hidden soy protein.

- **ALKYD RESIN SOLUTION:** Alkyd resin solution is made with soy oil, and is used in the creation of paint, cosmetics, toiletries and other household products.

- **QUATERNARY AMMONIUM SALTS:** Quaternary ammonium is a disinfectant that is used in many industrial and home applications; It is important to remember that if you are severely allergic to soy that the allergen can affect you through topical, skin contact just as much as through ingestion.

- **QUATERNARY AMMONIUM COMPOUNDS:** Soy based disinfectants made with soy oil.

- **ETHYLDIMETHYL SOYA ALKYL:** An extraction of soy oil; used as a disinfectant.

- **ET SOYETHYLDIMONIUM ETHOSULFATE:** Just one of an almost limitless variety of quaternary ammonium compounds used in industrial and home cleaning chemical products.

- **ALKYD RESIN:** Disinfectant, surfactant; part of a long chain of products deriving from soybean oil.

- **LINSEED OIL:** Linseed oil is often not 100% linseed oil with soybean oil being added to it in the manufacturing process. Linseed oil is traditionally rendered from flax. There is a food version, (flax oil), and an industrial version, (boiled linseed oil).

- **POLYMER PENTAERYTHRITOL:** Another in an endless variety of chemical derivatives both animal and vegetable based, usually soy, for use in paints, stains, and other industrial products.

- **PHTHALIC ANHYDRIDE:** Phthalic anhydride is a form of phthalic acid, used in the production of plastics, paints, dyes and many other industrial applications; a form of it is also used in the pharmaceutical industry as an enteric coating on medications and supplements. Exposure can cause symptoms that will mimic the flu.

- **STYRENE:** Styrene is mainly used in the

production of rubbers and plastics, and can indicate the presence of soy.

- **MORPHOLINIUM COMPOUNDS:** Morpholinium Compounds are a series of soy derivatives that have several industrial applications.

- **SOYAETHYL MORPHOLINIUM ETHOSULFATE:** You will find this chemical listed in the labels of many cosmetic products.

- **SOYATRIMONIUM CHLORIDE:** A soy derivative used in the toiletries and cosmetics industries as an antistatic, emulsifier, preservative, surfactant, (wetting agent), and as a conditioner.

- **TRIMETHYLSOYA:** Soy derivative used in toiletries and cosmetics industries.

- **VINYLTOLUENE:** A chemical solvent used in many industrial applications. It is a hydrocarbon similar to benzene.

- **ALKYL CHLORIDES:** Alkyl chlorides have been used in many industrial products.

- **QUATERNIUM-9:** Used in toiletries and skincare products.

- **POLYETHYLENE GLYCOL (PEG): PEG 5; PEG10; PEG 16; PEG 25; PEG 30; PEG 40 (SOY STEROLS):**
Usually soy-based chemical preparations used in toiletries, make-up and skincare products.

- **STEARIC ACID, STEARIC:** In terms of food products, stearic acid is used in making candy and supplements; this fatty acid is primarily used to produce cosmetics, soaps, and detergents. Stearic acid or stearic are definite signal terms for hidden soy. Be cautious if you see these terms in the label. See magnesium stearate below.

- **ISOSTEARYL ISOSTEARATE:** Used as binder and emollient in cosmetics. It is made from alcohols and vegetable fatty acids.

- **MAGNESIUM STEARATE:**
Magnesium stearate is rendered from soy. It is used in infant formulas, in powders and as a coating on certain candies, capsules, tablets, and supplements. Another place to find magnesium stearate is your bathtub; that accumulated matter called 'soap scum' is magnesium stearate.

- **TYRAMINE:** Tyramine is a natural amino acid that occurs in soy and many other foods.

- **UNO-HANA:** Uno-Hana is the Japanese term for soy pulp.

- **ISOLATED VEGETABLE PROTEIN:** Isolated vegetable protein is one of three main derivatives of soy, along with oil and what is called okara. Vegetable protein is a meat substitute or meat analogue; it is also added as filler to stretch other products purely for economics; it is even added to meat to form a hybrid product. That is why in a lot of cases the burger from your favorite fast food place will have soy indicated in both the meat and the bread.

- **METHYL CELLULOSE:** Methyl cellulose is a powder derived from vegetable cellulose. The odd property of methyl cellulose is that it can only be dissolved in cold water, not hot. When dissolved in water it becomes a gel that is used in cosmetics, toiletries, food products, and medicines as an emulsifier and thickener. It is purported to give foods a smoother, more appealing appearance.

- **PROTEIN FILLER:** Protein filler is another listing on food labels that will almost certainly indicate the presence of the soy allergen.

- **DIGLYCERIDES:** Diglycerides are fatty acids which act as emulsifiers in foodstuff; diglycerides often indicate the presence of soy. Contact the manufacturer, and read labels carefully. Most with a soy allergy can tolerate diglyceride with no ill effects.

- **MONO-DIGLYCERIDES:** Glycerides can come from animal or vegetable sources. They are simply fatty acids that are used as emulsifiers or blenders in food products— baked goods, ice cream, anything that needs a bridge between water and oil. They don't serve a major purpose in food production other than that, and probably should be avoided on that simple basis alone, being not very friendly fatty acids. But for the allergy sufferer, soy and otherwise, the problem comes into play if the diglyceride source is vegetable oil; the simple fact being that the vegetable oil is, more often than not, soy. For that specific reason, the soy allergy sufferer should read labels carefully, and if in doubt avoid any foods that contain mono-diglyceride. Our family has found that if mono-diglyceride is the only potential soy product listed, it is tolerable for a soy free diet. Every person has a different trigger level; it should be emphasized repeatedly that you are the captain of your own ship, and you must do what's right for you.

- **MONOTRIGLYCERIDE:** Mono-triglyceride is a fatty acid that is used as an additive in many foods. Glycerides can come from vegetable sources, soy being a main source; read labels carefully and contact the manufacturer to get further information.

- **GLYCOLS:** Glycols serve as solvents and as carriers for artificial/natural flavorings and colorings, as thickeners, as clarifiers and as stabilizers in mass produced, commercially processed foodstuffs. They are also used as preservatives: They are used in dressings; in soft drinks; in fat-free ice cream; in sour cream; in cake mixes. Their presence in a food product will in turn reveal the presence of soy.

- **TOCOTRETRIENOLS:** Tocotretrienols are derivatives that are a part of soy based make-up, and skincare products; if your soy allergy includes a sensitivity to topical products, you would need to avoid them.

- **SORBITAN TRISTEARATE:** Soy can be present in a wide range of products-- edibles, cosmetics, toiletries, cleaners, and disinfectants. Sorbitan Tristearate is a combination of fatty acids and natural sugar sterols that are derived from fruits like apples and pears; the fat particles can come from animal, nut and soy sources; if you note emulsifier, stearate, glycerides, glycols listed on labels, then your safest assumption is that the allergen is present.

I have attempted here to give as comprehensive a list as possible of both obvious and hidden soy products. As you can see that list is fairly long. To make sure that I don't mislead you entirely, I want to reemphasize that not all of these products will present a barrier. The difference between the allergenic qualities of proteins and oils is notable for most allergy sufferers. Many people with soy allergy can tolerate oil derivatives with no problems or side-effects whatsoever. It might be a little confusing to talk about all of these products as if they're all lumped together into one big mass; they're not of course. To go over it again to be clear: There are only two types of soy products—those derived from protein and those derived from oils. If you drew the family tree of soy, you would find more offspring on the oil side than on the protein side, but it is the protein that is the main culprit in an allergy. That does not mean that the oil isn't a problem. That is also why being a staunch captain of your own body ship is very, very, very important. If you are in doubt about any product, don't eat that product. I have provided lists in the appendices to help give a better picture of the breakdown of the different kinds of products and what soy derivatives might be present in them.

CHAPTER SEVEN
WHAT CAN I EAT?

To this point we've looked at the history of soy, and we've looked at the absolute mountain of soy products, the results of which reveal to us that soy is everywhere, and there are many processed foods that we can't eat. We've looked at what can happen if we accidentally or on a wild splurge eat something with soy, and how we need to be prepared for any circumstance. We've looked at some key areas where we need to be on guard, more conscious of our lifestyle choices and to make changes in the interest of managing a food allergy. So, hopefully at this point you can say with great assurance that you know what you shouldn't eat; that's good, but you also naturally want to know what you can safely eat. That's the question...

What Can I Eat?

A food allergy isn't the end of the world, and there is still a large variety of wonderful foods you can eat.

#

By now it sounds like a broken record, but deserves repeating: You have to think in terms of raw, fresh, whole, real, organic, (no additives), minimally processed, creative involvement—these become your new rallying points, your new watchwords. Managing your allergy may mean learning some new cooking skills, giving up a favorite food, patiently researching online, and methodically exploring the neighborhood to find out what's available in your community. It may mean ending a reliance on eating out so much, and definitely fast food joints, (cold reality—fast food doesn't seem to care about your allergy—to anything). We're going to go over fast food a little to give you an idea of what's available, and it's not expansive; I'm sorry if that dashes you. In terms of eat in restaurants, it's always an eye-opener to walk into a restaurant and ask about an allergy policy; in a lot of cases, you would find that there isn't anything formally established regarding how to safely serve people with a dangerous food allergy. There are some indications that this is changing, but it has been slow in coming.

As consumers we have to face the reality that we can't wean ourselves completely from the large chain distributors of our food; sadly we all can't become organic farmers, but that's the price we pay for convenience. What may have happened in the tradeoff is that we gave the food producers too much power over what we eat and how we eat. To take some of that power back we have to educate ourselves about how others are fiddling with and altering our food supply, in most cases just to make an extra buck. Allergy sufferers can be at the vanguard of a movement to make others aware of the need to be more conscious of how we needlessly play with our health and well-being and hopefully make a collective stand against all of the unhealthy tinkering with our food. We need to stop viewing our food as an industrial project and renew our view of it as a natural, sustaining force.

What can you eat? I'll go over it with as much depth as I can in the following pages so that you can get a full picture of where you stand in relationship to your allergy, and where you might need to make the most adjustment to eat safely and well. You can eat most everything; you just have to learn how to eat differently and more consciously—something all of us should learn how to do. The best idea is to simply take the recognized food groups, which are grains, dairy and eggs, fruits, vegetables, meats and proteins, oils and fats, and organize our exploration that way. Let's take a look:

BREADS:

You can eat breads, but as a note, most of what I will call shelf breads—the name brand breads you will find on the open grocery shelf—will contain soy flour, so your bread source will have to be specialty stores, or you can try making it yourself. Some people might find home bread-making adventurous, but most don't have time; have no fear, there are many wonderful bread sources out there.

* Look for whole flour
* Look for regular, self-rising
* Look for whole grain
* Look for alternatives, such as rice flour
* Look for any natural, allergy aware sources for bread you can find in your community; if you can't find it in your local vicinity, it might be worth a short drive to stock up on your bread, (if you can find it fairly close by), freeze it, and you'll have it ready when you want it. Panera Bread is a good source for some allergy friendly items; Whole Foods, the larger grocery stores always have specialty sections that will have some soyfree bakery items. You can always order it online:
* http://www.beckmannsbakery.com/
* http://daveskillerbread.com/breads/
* www.rudisbakery.com

What about Starches? There are lots of good things here to eat, with a few conditions:

- If you want mashed potatoes, you should cook **whole potatoes**, and mash them yourself because the bulk of instant potato flake brands contain soy, believe it or not. Better yet, check it out. There are a few that are soyfree if you can find them and if you just have to have the convenience. Give yourself a chance, before you graft those same old habits back onto extraordinary circumstances, to stop and connect with the spiritual and very simple, rewarding process of preparing and cooking food for yourself and your loved ones; there really isn't anything like the warm feeling of enjoying good food that you haven't poured out of a box, added some water to, presto, done, and as a healthy bonus, doesn't have a bunch of unnecessary additives.
- If you want french fries, make sure they are prepared in an oil other than soy oil.
- You can usually eat plain potato chips, but the flavored ones can contain soy in some form so read the labels carefully. Lay's has some soyfree products.
- Eat **sweet potatoes, yams**; they're good
- **Rice**: The plain instant varieties should be okay—make sure to check the labels—and whole plain rice, but avoid the flavored box dinner and side dish varieties; they're laden

with soy, usually. Rice is good protein, too.
- **Corn meal** is good as long as it isn't some kind of mix. Jiffy has some soyfree items.
- **Bread crumbs and batters**: look carefully at the ingredients before you buy anything; a lot of them have soy.
- **Pastas** can be a good protein source, and good for you in moderation.

What about other grains and cereals? You can eat them, and there is a lot of variety here:

- **Oatmeal, plain:** The instant flavored ones contain soy for the most part, and should generally be avoided; read labels, explore, and you may find a brand that is soyfree.
- **Grains** come in great abundant variety; explore them all, and build a renewed relationship with multi-grains. I won't name them all, but a small sampling follows:
  - Amaranth
  - Barley
  - Buckwheat Berries
  - Bulgur
  - Farro
  - Kamut
  - Long-grain Brown Rice
  - Millet
  - Oat Groats
  - Polenta
  - Popcorn
  - Quinoa, (So as not to offend, quinoa

is technically a seed, not a grain; it's good for you whatever its name).

- Red Quinoa, (Seed, not grain)
- Rye
- Short-grain Brown Rice
- Sorghum
- Spelt
- Sweet Brown Rice
- Teff
- Rolled Triticale
- Wheat Berries
- Wild Rice
- And many more

You can find these as flours, or use them as side dishes, hot cereals, or salads; they're very versatile, and have many health benefits.

VEGETABLES:

- Definitely get your full recommended servings of **vegetables**; in connection with your soy allergy, you want to apply one of those magic watchwords outlined above— **FRESH**. You want to gravitate toward fresh vegetables as much as possible.
- There are canned varieties that you can find with a little digging that will be preserved with just salt and water, but they are few. A note here: some of the store brands are better at presenting more soy free foods than name brands.

FRUIT:

- **FRESH fruits** definitely need to be at the top of your grocery list.
- There are some **frozen WHOLE varieties** that are good to go if they are just the fruit, and no other additives; the fruits sold for making smoothies are really good, and are usually just the fruit.
- With a little searching you can find some canned fruits that are soyfree as well.
- Most canned fruit pie fillings are soyfree, too; look at labels carefully to be sure.
- Dried Fruits: most are safe; make sure to read the labels.
- Don't forget **apricots** and **peaches**; they're surprisingly high in protein, believe it or not.

BEVERAGES:

- **Soda, pop, soft drinks**: There are other reasons not to drink soda of any kind, but I'll leave that to your discretion; in terms of soy allergy, however, they are safe to use. A lot of the energy, power drinks do have soy.
- **Water**; be careful of flavored waters, and water flavor packets; most of them contain soy, but a few don't. Read labels and do your research.
- **Teas:** Use caution. Some blends have soy.

- **Coffee, plain**; but be careful of the special coffees; most of the flavored coffees and blends contain soy.
- **Single fruit juices** are usually good; be wary of concentrates, juice blends, and other indicators like ade, cocktail—those will, in most cases, contain soy.

MEAT AND MEAT SUBSTITUTES:

- **Fresh beef**
- **Fresh chicken**
- **Fresh lamb**
- **Fresh pork**
- **Fresh turkey**
- **Fresh veal**
- **Fresh Fish and other seafood**
- **Frozen varieties** of all of these can be eaten as long as they come without prebasting, rubs, gravies, sauces, or prebreading; you can always make your own.
- **Deli meats** are a gray area because often you can't get a clear answer about what they contain; they're good to go if you know there aren't any additives in the form of protein fillers, or products used for coloring and flavor. A meat extender in the form of textured vegetable protein is often used in commercially produced meat like luncheon loaf, ham loaf, sausages and hot dogs.
- **Seaweed**, high protein source; **spirulina** is the supplement version.

- **Seitan** is another food to try; let's call it wheat tofu. Called mock duck sometimes, It's actually wheat gluten formed into a paste that is then treated like tofu.
- **Tree nuts**; that includes **coconut**.

MILK AND MILK PRODUCTS:

- **Whole milk and skimmed varieties**; check flavored milks carefully; they can contain soy. Be careful of what are called filled milks, (skim milk/condensed milk, with vegetable oil added back in to raise the fat content).
- **Yogurt**, mostly plain: You can always add your own fruits and natural flavorings if you know where they came from. A lot of the flavored varieties are soyfree as well.
- **Real 100% cheese;** artificial varieties most times contain soy; you can find some that don't.
- **Cottage cheese;** read the labels to make sure there are no soy ingredients in it.
- **Cream Cheese:** Most are safe; read the labels anyway.
- **Sour Cream:** Most should be alright; check to be sure.
- **Eggs:** Whole eggs are 100% safe; mixed, dietetic versions, maybe not so safe. Check labels carefully.

SOUPS AND COMBINATION FOODS:

- **Make your own;** it's fun and tastes better too. You will find as you explore, read labels, and start to rearrange your diet to accommodate the soy allergen that most prepared, fully processed, pre-packaged, combination foodstuffs, either in cans or in the refrigerated sections of the stores will contain soy. There are some that don't, but you WILL have to search to find them; that is also dependent on the severity of your allergy. As stated before, some have no problem with soy oil, and can enjoy foods that have only that as the soy related additive. Don't experiment indiscriminately; remember, if in doubt, avoid it.

DESSERTS AND SWEETS:

- **Ice Cream:** Read the labels; a lot of brands add soy.
- **Cookies, pastries, snack cakes, cakes:** You can eat these, but you need to look for soyfree versions or make your own. The frostings for cakes also have soy, so be careful there, too. Read the labels, read the labels, read the labels.
- **Puddings, the boiled kind.** Most of the other varieties will have soy.

FATS AND OILS:

You can safely use—in context of the allergen--the following oils:

- **Avocado oil**—Avocado oil is billed to have the highest smoke point of any other vegetable oil. It is an excellent, all round healthy oil, but it can be very expensive. The 16.9 oz version costing around $16.00.
- **Canola oil**—canola oil has been in the news lately as a potentially unsafe oil: a new development requiring more study.
- **Coconut oil**—You can't go wrong with coconut oil. It's a good old standard, been around a long time, with a good, healthy track record.
- **Corn oil**—Your basic vegetable oil.
- **Flax seed oil**—Very healthy, a good cooking oil.
- **Grapeseed oil**—A good cooking oil, but very expensive.
- **Olive oil**—Olive oil is good for you, but may not be the best choice for all foods because of the strong taste factor. It is also very expensive.
- **Palm oil**—The getting of the oil is not very friendly for the environment, and some grocery stores have begun to ban it from the shelves, but there are sustainable versions around; you have to do a little extra digging. Something to keep in mind.

- **Peanut oil**—be cautious of this one as it could be an associative allergen.
- **Safflower oil**—A basic, good alternative.
- **Sesame oil**—Not so much for cooking, but great for making salad dressings.
- **Sunflower oil**—Once again can't go wrong here, good old standby.
- **Walnut oil**—Very good all-purpose cooking oil, healthy, but expensive.

CAUTIONARY NOTE; the label must indicate a specific oil so that you know what you're getting, or it is suspect, and you should avoid it. For example: If the label says VEGETABLE OIL with no other information, choose another oil.

- **REAL BUTTER:** Most margarines contain some form of soy product.
- **Shortening**—there are specialty versions; look for them in the natural, organic, specialty sections of your store.

CONDIMENTS AND MISCELLANEOUS FOODS:

- Regular sugar
- Splenda
- Stevia
- Truvia
- Artificial sweeteners
- Salt
- Pepper
- Whole spices; be careful of spice blends,

and mixes, or avoid completely
- Jane's Krazy Mixed-up Salt is okay
- Use **Canola mayonnaise**, or you may find other base oils as well. There is also a **safflower mayonnaise**.
- Use a **soy sauce substitute**. There is a delicious one made with coconut.
- **Salad dressings are difficult**; it takes some exploration, or you can **make your own**—they're usually simple and easy to whip together.

These condiments are pretty much all safe; read labels anyway.

- Ketchup
- Mustard
- Pickles and Relishes
- Honey
- Molasses or organic blackstrap molasses
- Jams and Jellies
- Syrup or organic maple syrup
- Plain Sugar Candies
- Powdered Cocoa
- 100% Dark Baker's Chocolate; chocolate and desserts in general are one of the biggest problem areas in relation to coping with the allergen. Relax, don't cry. You can still have chocolate. You just have to go a little further out on Willie Wonka's chocolate tree limb to get it.

WHAT ABOUT FAST FOOD?

I had no notion of the number of fast food eateries there were out there until I began my research for this book; there are hundreds of them, and they have proliferated like weeds over the years, and now you can find one on every corner and throughway of everywhere even in the smallest towns. You may not be able to find specialty breads anywhere in your hometown, but it's guaranteed that you will find a McDonalds, or some other of that ilk, you fill in the blank. Guess What? They're soy factories!

#

If you have developed a soy allergy and you are in the habit of grabbing a quick bite for lunch, or you like the food for whatever reason, here is an area where your life will change. You won't be able to dash out to your local favorite fast food 'restaurant' without some extra deliberation. Fast food establishments are not very accommodating to people with any kind of allergy, if that's of any consolation to you. It's not some evil conspiracy, it's just economic considerations plus the catering to the lowest common denominator of consumer, the default eater. I thought we'd get the bad news out of the way first.

The somewhat good news is that you can find things to eat at all of those places; if you like salad without the dressing, (practically all dressings will have soy in them), you're in good territory, and if you like your burger minus the meat patty, (most of them have vegetable protein extenders in them), and the bun, (most of them have soy in them), then chow down. In the interest of not painting an impossible picture of fast food, you can still eat at your favorite restaurant, it's just that post allergy confirmation, your choices will be definitely limited to a few items on each menu that fortunately may not have soy somewhere in the mix. The most important thing to understand is that you won't be able to order anything you like as may have been the case before. It will be a salad here, chicken nuggets there, kid's burger somewhere else, a plain piece of fried fish at another, grilled somethings at different places. It's scattered pickings, and slim pickings.

Another important consideration, and this is where you need to be proactive, and weigh your options in terms of maybe completely changing your eating habits—all of those fast food items use the same production, finishing lines, and those non-soy items will be mixed in with the soy items. Whether that affects you or not depends on the severity of your allergy and the history of your reactions to the allergen. Some people react severely to the oil, and others it doesn't affect. In general, the restaurants will be following the FDA standards in both food handling and food preparation, and the FDA doesn't consider soy oil a causal agent, only soy protein. You are in control of you, and only you know if you can take a chance on food prepared outside your control and supervision. Remember the cardinal rule, if in doubt, avoid the food. A burger isn't worth a hospital trip.

I want to get radical here for a short time. If I had to choose sides in a debate about whether or not fast food is good or bad on some scale, I would fall somewhere on the bad side. In other words, there is more to be aware of in terms of potential dangers of fast food than the fact that it is laden with soy across the board; why not, it's cheap, and goes a long way through the food lines. We're focusing on soy here, but when you add in all of the other bugaboos related to fast food, it makes you wonder if anyone should eat fast food, at all, ever again. This may not get me any perks with the fast food purveyors out there, but quite frankly I care more about us than I do about them. I won't extend my tirade here, but suffice it to say that we have a lot of work to do to clean up our nutritional act.

What we call fast food is a strange mix of this and that; it's really hard to define in terms of what is and isn't fast food, and the demarcation line is hard to establish. I use service as a divider: If there is a dedicated server who brings your food to you after you order it at a table, it stops being fast food. I don't know if that holds up, but it's my personal measure. In terms of poor or even bad nutritional value, then fast food extends into infinity. On the other hand, it could be said that any food prepared in a commercial setting, i.e., food you didn't prepare for yourself at home, is suspect for both nutrition and safety as it relates to the allergen.

The wild thing about an allergy is that it forces you to look at food overall, and you start to see that there is more than just the allergen that is wrong with food, especially what can be termed professional hospitality food. You start to see, become more curious about and begin to develop a desire to define all of those unpronounceable, unnecessary items that get tossed into our food, and the shock grows, and you start to wonder why in hell is there carmine in my food. Carmine, in case anyone is wondering, is a red food dye rendered from the body of a species of beetle. By the way, if you've ever ordered a strawberry drink, you've ingested carmine—just a small sampling for your edification.

To help a little, I'm going to relate a few things about the restaurants themselves, but I'm not going to go over each one methodically; not only would that take forever, but it would be a volume in and of itself. Each chain has an online presence and most do offer separate sites, either pdf charts or online interactive apps, where you can get complete nutritional information on each item in their menu along with the allergens that may be present. I will catalog those for your convenience, but I won't talk about the foods; I'll rather give an overview and you can research and explore from there: It's an eye-opener in some cases relative to where you will find soy. To preface a bit further, and to give some credit, a number of fast food establishments are starting to make tentative efforts to clean up their nutritional act by removing allergens and also lowering bad fats and such, so there is hope, a little.

#

Here are some general elements to consider; please understand that these are not hard facts, merely observations that came from looking at data:

- The more dine in, direct service at table features are emphasized, the more possibilities there will be for soyfree menu items, and allergy friendly accommodations overall; this isn't based on science, merely elementary observation.
- The more preparation choices you have, the greater your chances are of finding some soyfree items.
- The more the establishment focuses on branded products, the more limited the soyfree items.
- The greater the variety of food overall, the better your chances are of finding soyfree foods.

All of the above are generalizations based on an examination of data, and don't represent any hard and fast rules; always do your own research so that you can effectively manage your soy allergy. Below is a list of some of those many restaurants with their websites so you can check out their ingredients and nutritional listings for yourself. Some don't seem to have chosen to post allergy specific guides, and in those cases I have included the base website so you can do your own sleuthing. The chains always have a telephone contact listing; don't be afraid or embarrassed to call and ask questions, get the answers you need. It is hoped that representatives would know what is in the food they serve. It is serious if they don't:

- **A & W—**
  http://www.awrestaurants.com/Allergens%20&%20Sensitivities%20Grid.pdf

- **Applebee's—**
  http://www.applebees.com/~/media/docs/Applebees_Allergen_Info.pdf

- **Arby's—**
  http://cds.arbys.com/pdfs/nutrition/USMenuItems_Ingrdnts_JAN.pdf

- **Baja Fresh—**
  http://www.bajafresh.com/mexican-food-nutrition

- **Baker's Drive Through—**
  http://www.bakersdrivethru.com/nutritional-info/

- **Baskin Robbins**—Allergy line is 800-859-5339

- **Big Boy**—http://www.bigboy.com

- **Blimpie**—
http://www.blimpie.com/assets/pdf/
BlimpieAllergensChart.pdf

- **Bojangles**—
http://www.bojangles.com/_assets/pdf/B
OJ_Nutrition_Facts_2013.pdf

- **Boston Pizza**—
http://www.bostonpizza.com

- **Burger King**—there's an online interactive menu or get a PDF version with nutritional and allergy information included. It's hard to read, so be prepared to spend a little time checking everything out and making comparisons.

- **Carl's Jr.**--
http://www.carlsjr.com/system/pdf_menu
s/3/original/CJ_GB_Allergen_Chart_01.10.
14.pdf?1389396524

- **Checkers**—http://www.checkers.com

- **Chick-Fil-A**—Click on Food tab, then on Health and Allergen information.

- **Chipotle**—http://www.chipotle.com/en-us/menu/special_diet_information/special_diet_information.aspx ✶ ✶ ✶ ✶ ✶

- **Chuck E. Cheese's**—Download from their site by state and location.

- **Church's Chicken**—http:www.churchs.com

- **Cold Stone Creamery**—http://www.coldstonecreamery.com/assets/pdf/nutrition/cold-stone-creamery-allergen_chart.pdf

- **Culver's**—http://culvers-bece73af.s3.amazonaws.com/page-content/menu/CulversAllergenBrochure.pdf

- **Dagwoods**—http://www.dagwoodssandwiches.com

- **Dairy Queen**—http://www.dairyqueen.com/Documents/2013NutritionFoodTreatUS_Revised.pdf

- **Denny's**—http://dennys.com/files/Allergen_PamphletMarch2013.pdf

- **Domino's Pizza**—https://order.dominos.com/en/pages/cont

ent/nutritional/allergen-info.jsp

- **Dunkin Donuts—**
  http://www.dunkindonuts.com/
  content/dunkindonuts/en/
  menu/nutrition/nutrition_catalog.html?
  nutrition_cat

- **El Pollo Loco—**http://www.elpolloloco.com

- **Fat Burger—**
  http://www.fatburger.com/PDF/FBR8_Alle
  rgens_M1.pdf

- **Fazoli's**--
  http://www.fazolis.com
  https://s3.amazonaws.com/desktop_assets
  /fazolis/menu/ingredient_statement.pdf

- **Five Guys Burgers and Fries—**
  http://www.fiveguys.com

- **Fuddruckers—**
  http://www.fuddruckers.com/

- **Hardee's—**
  http://www.hardees.com/system/pdf_men
  us/13/original/H_RB_Allergen_Chart_Cove
  r_2013.pdf?1384455321

- **Hooters—**http://www.hooters.com

- **IHOP—**
  http://www.ihop.com/-/media/ihop/PDFs
  /allergeninformation.ashx

- **Jack in the Box—**
  http://assets.jackinthebox.com/pdf_attach
  ment_settings/107/value/Allergen_Referen
  ce_Guide.pdf

- **Jamba Juice—**http://jambajuice.com

- **Johnny Rockets—**
  http://www.johnnyrockets.com/menu/alle
  rgen-alert.html

- **Kentucky Fried Chicken—**
  http://www.kfc.com/nutrition/pdf/kfc_alle
  rgens.pdf

- **Krispy Kreme—**
  http://www.krispykreme.com/about-
  us/nutritional-information

- **Krystal—**http://www.krystal.com

- **Licks Homeburgers and Ice Cream**--
  http://lickshomeburgers.com

- **Little Caesars—**
  http://www.littlecaesars.com

- **Long John Silvers—**

http://www.ljsilvers.com/images/pdfs/LJS
_Customer_Ingredient_List_January_2014.p
df

- **McDonalds—**
  http://nutrition.mcdonalds.com/
  getnutrition/ingredientslist.pdf

- **Miami Subs Pizza and Grill—**
  http://www.miamisubs.com

- **MR SUB**—http://www.mrsub.com

- **Nathan's Famous—**
  http://www.nathansfamous.com

- **New York Fries—**
  http://www.newyork fries.com

- **Orange Julius—**
  http://www.dairyqueen.com/
  Documents/OJ%20Nutrition
  %202013%20US_October.pdf

- **Papa Gino's Pizza—**
  http://www.papaginos.com

- **Papa John's Pizza—**
  http://www.papajohns.com/about/
  papa-johns-ingredients.shtm

- **Pizza Donini**—http://www.doninis.com

- **Pizza Hut**—http://www.pizzahut.com/foodallergies.html

- **Popeye's Chicken and Biscuits**—http://popeyes.com/menu/nutrition

- **Quizno's Sub**—Great allergy aware site; the **interactive allergy guide** is a great feature. You can also download an allergen grid as a pdf.

- **Rally's**—http://rallys.com/pdf/nutritional_information.pdf

- **Red Lobster**—http://www.redlobster.com/health/allergy/pdf/RL_Allergen_Menu.pdf

- **Red Robin**—Red Robin, too has a great **interactive allergy guide** that can be used anywhere.

- **Roy Rogers Family Restaurants**—http://www.royrogersrestaurants.com

- **Sbarro**—http://www.sbarro.com

- **Sonic**--http://sonicwww.s3.amazonaws.com/Content/pdfs/Sonic_Allergen_Table.pdf

- **South Street Burger Company—** http://www.southstburger.com

- **Subway—** http://www.subway.com/Nutrition/Files/US_Allergen_chart.pdf

- **Taco Bell** http://www.tacobell.com/nutrition/allergens

- **Taco Bueno—**http://www.tacobueno.com

- **Taco Tico—**http://www.tacotico.com

- **Tim Hortons—** http://www.timhortons.com/us/pdf/Allergen_Information_-_USA_-_December2013.pdf

- **Wendy's—** http://www.wendys.com/redesign/wendys/pdf/en_US_nutrition.pdf

- **Whataburger—** http://www.whataburger.com

- **White Castle—** http://www.whitecastle.com/nutrition

- **Zaxby's—** http://www.zaxbys.com/menu_nutrition/allergen_information.aspx?AllID=6

MORE THOUGHTS ON FAST FOOD

To give an idea of the prevalence of soy in fast food environments, let's approach it not from brands but from the notion of key words:

- **Bun**—Count on the buns that sandwich fast food branded products to have soy. That's the majority of the time.

- **Burger**—Anytime you see the word burger on the menu, there will be soy, primarily in the bun, but a lot of times in the meat too.

- **Dressing**—Sometimes you will run across a dressing without soy proteins added, but it is rare. Your hope is vinaigrette, but make sure of what the oil is before you eat it if you respond negatively to the oil as well as the protein.

- **Breaded**—If you see this word, there will be soy in most cases. The allergy sheets can give you more targeted information.

- **Sauce**—Pretty much all sauces will have soy products.

- **Mayonnaise**—mayonnaise is made with soy oil; there are, as we've learned, a few alternatives, but it isn't likely that even one restaurant will stock them. They're very expensive.

- **Fried, fries**—in the majority of times, a fried food in a restaurant will be cooked in generic vegetable oil, which is more likely than not, soybean oil.

- **Chocolate**—Everything included here from chocolate milkshakes, the chocolate drizzle on desserts, chocolate chips. Soy lecithin is usually the additive here.

- **Glaze**—special glazes for meats, especially, will have soy proteins in them.

- **Margarine**—unless it's real butter it will have soy in it.

- **Cheese**—largest percentage of likelihood, you can count on the cheese, including both sauces and slices, having soy.

- **Cookies**—pretty much all varieties of baked goos will have soy.

- **Pies**—both the fillings and the crust will have soy.

- **Biscuits**—breakfast food will have soy in some form.

- **Gravy**—breakfast gravy will contain soy.

- **Pizza dough**—Largest percent of products. This can change so continue to monitor and check the listings.

- **Pizza toppings**—will contain soy, mainly protein additives in the largest percentage of situations, and across the spectrum of fast food providers of pizza products.

- **Coffee**—the highly flavored, blended coffees will have soy.

- **Ice Cream**—ice cream in most instances will have soy additives.

CHAPTER EIGHT
HOW TO READ
FOOD LABELS

The Food and Drug Administration requires foods that contain or may contain any amount of egg, milk, fish, shellfish, peanut, nuts, wheat and soy, the top eight allergy causing foods be indicated on the label. Some labels are clearly marked, but there are hidden ingredients and those ingredients are what you need to look for carefully before you buy.

Sometimes labels specifically say CONTAINS SOY INGREDIENTS—this is required by law; at other times you will see ALLERGY WARNING: CONTAINS MILK AND WHEAT. MAY CONTAIN TRACES OF EGG AND SOY. There are other variations in these required warnings. In these cases, the information is precise and easy to understand. It is the information regarding hidden ingredients that can create problems for the allergy sufferer.

Since 2006, after the Food Allergen and Consumer Protection Act (FALCPA) became law, food manufacturers have been required to list what is in prepared foods, though they are not required to reveal to the consumer the full origin of a product. Let's take mono-diglycerides for example: you will see diglycerides listed in the ingredients, but you won't see a notation they are obtained from soy. In practically every case, it is a sure and safe bet to assume that mono-diglycerides are soy based and most allergy sufferers should avoid any food products with that designator. While mono-diglycerides are not high on the list of worries, it would be nice to know if the source was soy so that the soy allergy sufferer can make a more informed decision. Hopefully at some point, that will be changed, but for now the labeling standards are still in a state of flux and ongoing development.

WHAT'S THE DIFFERENCE BETWEEN 'CONTAINS' AND 'MAY CONTAIN'?

Furthermore what does 'and/or' mean relative to reading food labels? Pointedly, we don't know exactly what it means—you will see this in relation to oils; contains palm oil and/or soy oil.

That's wonderful of them to inform us, but we still don't know what the situation is in that case. The only way to find out is to contact the producer and ask. Which is it? Is it both? Is it one or the other; if it is, which one is it because if it's palm oil, buy it, take it home and enjoy it, and if it's soy it would be better to exercise caution and not use it, dependent on the severity of your allergy?

Okay then: What is the difference between contains and may contain? On the one hand, you can be certain to avoid the product so labeled, but with the latter you can be fairly certain that it is best for you to avoid it as well, but it doesn't really help in the long run because it creates a drop in communication that puts a burden on the consumer; we don't know why we're given the run around, but they, meaning producers and manufacturers, offer up the cursory explanations below regarding what it all means, somewhat in response to arbitrary labeling laws:

- **Contains** means that the product in question does definitely have soy as one of its ingredients, either as a direct soy by product or one of many derivatives. The decision is simple: Avoid the food that CONTAINS the target allergen.

- **May Contain** means (1) the food has soy as a slight percentage amount in a compound ingredient such as an oil mixture—different vegetable oils and soy oil are sometimes mixed, for example, and you won't know that if you don't ask or if it isn't labeled directly, (2) the food product was packaged or prepared in an area or on equipment where it may have become 'contaminated' by the allergen, and (3) it could be that a version of a product has soy while another doesn't—sometimes there are variations in different sizes of the same product. Another important thing to note about 'may contain' is that it is voluntary on the part of manufacturers. The consumer's decision-making isn't so simple: The only way to know if it is safe is to ask questions to get a definitive answer. The only certainty is to avoid that food altogether as well.

WHAT TO LOOK FOR:

Reading labels is one of the most important allergy management practices. The core list below will indicate the presence of soy if you note these products included on labels; you need to avoid products with these listings. More comprehensive lists are included, but this is a sampling of things to definitely look for:

- Edamame—soybean pods
- Hydrolyzed Soy Protein
- Kinnoko flour
- Kyodofu—freeze-dried tofu

- Miso—azuki bean miso, alternative
- Natto
- Okara—Soy pulp
- Shoyu Sauce
- Soy Albumin
- Soy Bran
- Soy Concentrate
- Soy Fiber
- Soy Flour
- Soy Formula
- Soy Grits
- Soy Milk—cow and almond milk, alternates
- Soy Miso
- Soy Nuts
- Soy Nut Butter
- Soy Protein, Soy Protein Concentrate, Soy Protein Isolate
- Soy sauce—coconut aminos, alternative
- Soy Sprouts—mung sprouts, alternative
- Soya, shoya
- Soya Flour
- Soybeans, Soybean Granules
- Soybean Curd
- Soybean Flour
- Soy Lecithin—In most cases you won't see soy lecithin listed, but if the product contains it, the label may say 'contains soy'.
- Soybean Paste
- Soy Oil
- Supro is soy protein isolate
- Tamari
- Tempeh

- Teriyaki Sauce
- Textured Soy Flour (TSF)
- Textured Soy Protein (TSP)
- Textured Vegetable Protein (TVP)
- Tofu—seitan, alternative
- Yakidofu
- Yuba—bean curd
- Vegetable Oil—Vegetable oil, even if it is soy based, you will see touted as safe for allergy sufferers; but from experience, it is best to apply the cardinal rule of avoidance if there is any doubt about how your system might react.

Other ingredients to look for that more likely than not indicates the presence of soy:

- Artificial Flavoring
- Asian foods—This is anything advertised as Japanese, Chinese, Thai, etc. NOTE: This is not to denigrate those cultures in any way; in this context, the safety of the allergy sufferer is most important.
- Diglycerides
- Hydrolyzed Plant Protein
- Hydrolyzed Vegetable Protein (HVP)
- Mono-diglycerides
- Natural Flavoring
- Vegetable Broth
- Vegetable Gum
- Vegetable Starch

Let's take a look at some random labels to get used to searching for a specific set of data, in this case soy; it's surprising where you will find soy hiding. In this section, I am deliberately refraining from identifying brands in relation to reading labels because it first of all doesn't matter as production methods and practices are pretty much standardized, and there are fewer soy-free products than there are ones that definitely contain soy ingredients. This isn't to imply that brands and companies have instituted some evil conspiracy against the soy allergy sufferer—it may imply an insensitivity—but it does imply that cost cutting and stretching measures have been implemented in the production process by the manufacturers; soy is very cheap. Secondly, we're not worried so much about any brand, but what the label is telling us is in a particular food; we need to concentrate on the ingredients, and we need to give up any brand name loyalties that we might have. The goal is to find good things that we can eat as allergy sufferers, not to promote brand following. Finally, all brands may have some wonderful products that are soy free that you can safely enjoy; you can only know that by reading labels.

#

Here are those labels at random to simply give a cross-section and provide practice with isolating and identifying ingredients; they are not in any specific order, and they cover everything from Worcestershire sauce to snack cakes; when you start reading labels, you'll see most of these ingredients everywhere, on almost every label:

WORCESTERSHIRE SAUCE:

A premier brand; does it contain soy?

- Ingredients: distilled white vinegar, molasses, water, sugar, onions, anchovies, salt, garlic, cloves, tamarind extract, natural flavorings, chili pepper extract. Contains anchovies.

The recipe is declared a secret, but by some reports Worcestershire contains soy derivatives. Though in looking at the ingredients as they are listed here, there isn't much evidence of soy. Unless there is some really hidden stuff, this one basically passes the test; the only potential indicator is the generic 'natural flavorings' listing, which could, and often does, reveal the presence of soy protein. The label will sometimes say Allergy warning: Contains anchovies, may contain traces of wheat and soy. Anyone with a known severe soy allergy should definitely avoid this product to be safe until you find out for certain that there isn't any hidden soy in it. Always best to apply the rule—if in doubt, avoid it.

FROSTED CHERRY POMEGRANATE TOASTER PASTRIES:

This one is a natural foods brand that my family

has used a lot; let's test this one. Does it contain soy?

- INGREDIENTS: Wheat flour*, evaporated cane juice invert*, evaporated cane juice*, palm oil*, cherries*, apples*, whole wheat flour*, corn starch*, vital wheat gluten*, sea salt, leavening (baking soda, cream of tartar), tapioca starch*, pomegranate juice concentrate*, dextrose*, rice starch*, cherry flavor*, citric acid, honey*, molasses*, rice bran extract*, vanilla flavor*, algin, sodium citrate, monocalcium phosphate, whey protein concentrate (milk)*, colored with betalains, paprika extract (from plants). *Organic. Contains wheat and dairy.

Yea, this one is soyfree, chow down! It's good! If you look carefully at the ingredients list, it's easy to see that this one is concentrated on using organic products, but that doesn't concern us—it shows food mindfulness and that's great—as much as the allergen. In this case it is free of soy allergen. A person allergic to wheat could not use this food, of course, but for a soy allergy it's good to go.

GLUTEN FREE CAKE MIX:

This is a well-known brand of yellow cake mix marketed as gluten free, hence the presence of xanthan gum, which possibly indicates the presence of soy in and of itself. The addition of the xanthan gum is necessary because the gluten has been removed:

- Ingredients: Rice Flour, sugar, Potato starch, Leavening (Baking Soda, Sodium Acid Pyrophosphate, monocalcium phosphate) Xanthan Gum, Salt. Gluten free. Gluten free. May contain soy ingredients. Do not eat raw cake batter.

This one is an almost, but probably not for soy allergy sufferers. The label says it may contain soy ingredients, which plants doubt in our mind. There are potential problems in the Xanthan Gum; soy, as well as other vegetables, can play host to the bacterium that yields Xanthan, and other than contacting the manufacturer to find out for sure there isn't any way to know. The thinking here is that we should assume it does contain soy in some form, and choose a different food. You can also read that xanthan gum is less of an allergen than other more direct soy derivatives, and can be tolerated with no side effects by the soy allergy sufferer. Only you ultimately know the extent of your allergy; you are in control, and always remember the key rule —if in doubt, don't use it.

SUPER MOIST CAKE MIX:

The very famous brand again with a super moist version cake mix. Is it soyfree? Let's look:

- Ingredients: Enriched Flour Bleached (Wheat Flour, Niacin, Iron, Thiamin Mononitrate, Riboflavin, Folic Acid) Sugar, Corn Syrup, Leavening (Baking Soda, Sodium Aluminum Phosphate, Monocalcium Phosphate), Contains 2% less of: Modified Corn starch, Corn starch, Partially Hydrogenated Soybean and/or cottonseed Oil, Propolene Glycol Mono and Diesters of Fatty Acids, salt, distilled Monoglycerides, dicalcium Phosphate, Natural and Artificial Flavor, sodium stearoyl Lactylate, Xanthan Gum, Cellulose Gum, Yellows 5 & 6, Nonfat Milk. Contains wheat and milk ingredients.

One important key piece of information that the allergy sufferer needs to keep as a mental note is that the labeling laws do not cover certain products, and some are exempt from labeling by the FDA because it's determined that they're not harmful such as soy oil. Those constitute the hidden products that are often talked about. This one, for safety's sake, should not be used on a soy free diet; there are several possible problems here: Soybean oil, xanthan gum, propylene glycol, mono-glycerides, natural and artificial flavor. The soybean oil is an and/or, and the others in most instances indicate a soy source. You could contact the manufacturer in this instance to inquire about these additives, but why not simply choose to be safe and leave it behind and choose a soyfree version. They are out there. You could also get adventurous and make your own.

PEANUT BUTTER CHEESE CRACKER SNACK SANDWICHES:

We call these nabs where I come from; they've appeared in more lunch boxes and vending machines than can be imagined perhaps, and it's impossible to count how many have been consumed. They're not very healthy, and everyone should leave them behind, but they are loved and favored and savored everywhere. They are 220 calories of unnecessary consumption, though it's undeniable—love the nabs, but are they soyfree?

- Ingredients: Enriched Wheat Flour (Containing Niacin, Reduced Iron, Thiamine Mononitrate, Riboflavin, Folic Acid, Peanuts, Vegetable Oil (Contains one or more of the following vegetable oils: Canola Oil, Corn Oil, Palm Oil, Soy Oil), Dextrose, Salt, Sugar, Leavening (Sodium Bicarbonate), Malted Barley Flour, Yeast, Cheddar Cheese (Cultured Pasteurized Milk, Salt, Enzymes), Artificial Color (Contains FD&C Yellow 6), Disodium Phosphate. Contains: wheat, milk, peanuts.

There is a possible presence of soy, though not as much as you might think, but because there is a mystery as to the oil, it might be best to err on the side of avoiding it, and opt for a product that is more clear about its constituents.

TUNA:

Several brands, same processing measures; Tuna doesn't contain soy, it's meat, seafood, right? Hmm!

- Ingredients: Light Tuna, Soybean Oil, Vegetable Broth (Contains Soy), Salt.

That's it! Those are the ingredients of this brand and indeed most brands. Who knew? Most canned meats do contain soy. This is a product that should not be a part of a soyfree diet under any circumstances. Fortunately, there are some brands out there that are soyfree; look for skipjack tuna with just water and salt.

PANCAKE AND BAKING MIX:

Once again, a famous brand, a household word actually, but we're not concentrating on brands; we're pretending everything's generic, and we're reading labels to determine if what we're planning to buy and use has soy; let's test this one, and get some more practice looking at labels:

- Ingredients: Enriched Flour bleached (wheat flour, niacin, iron, thiamin, mononitrate, riboflavin, folic acid), Partially Hydrogenated Soybean and/or Cottonseed Oil, Leavening (baking soda, sodium aluminum phosphate, monocalcium phosphate), Dextrose, Salt.

The potential allergen here is the soybean oil; once more the consumer is hit with that waffling and/or designator, and we are left with uncertainty. This probably should not be included in a soyfree diet because of the soybean oil. Some allergy sufferers can tolerate soybean oil, and the FDA does exempt soy oil from labeling standards, but in the case of any allergy, it is always, always better to be safe than sorry and avoid a questionable product altogether, especially since there are alternatives to this type of flour mix product; plus you can always cook from scratch.

VEGETABLE CLASSICS LENTIL SOUP:

A great soup from a company famous for soup; can a person with a soy allergy eat it? Let's read the label and find out:

- Ingredients: Water, Lentils, Celery, Tomato Paste, Modified Food Starch, Spinach. Contains less than 1% of: Salt, Soybean Oil, Sugar, Natural Flavor.

A grocery shopper looking at this might say to himself or herself-I can eat this because the indicated amounts of soy products are less than 1%. The problem with this: the concentration doesn't matter with some but it seriously matters with others; when it comes to the allergen, a minute amount can bring about unwanted side effects. We stated in another section that the allergy is keyed to amounts, but this can't always be relied on. An allergy is a mysterious thing; that is why you should always observe great caution in testing things out. The one soy product, and the potential soy product indicated by natural flavor help us to arrive at the best decision; the person with a soy allergy should avoid this one and choose a completely soyfree product. They are out there and don't require that much exploring to find them.

HONEY BUNS SNACK CAKES:

You know this brand; it's a household word. Does this product have soy in it?

- Ingredients: Enriched Bleached Flour (Wheat Flour, Barley Malt, Niacin, Reduced Iron, Thiamine Mononitrate, (Vitamin B1), Riboflavin (Vitamin B2), Folic Acid), Water, Sugar, Palm Oil, Partially Hydrogenated Soybean and Cottonseed Oil with TBHQ to Preserve Flavor (Contributes a Trivial Amount of Trans Fats), Dextrose, Yeast, Contains 2% or Less of Each of the Following: Soy Flour, Nonfat Dry Milk, Dried Honey, Eggs, Cinnamon, Cocoa, Wheat Starch, Partially Hydrogenated Soybean and/or Cottonseed Oil (Contributes a Trivial Amount of Trans Fats), Leavening (Baking Soda, Sodium Acid Pyrophosphate). Corn Starch, Soybean Oil, Salt, Calcium Stearoyl Lactylate, Calcium Carbonate, Agar, Emulsifiers (Datem, Mono and Diglycerides, soy Lecithin), calcium sulfate, calcium Propionate and Potassium Sorbate (to Retain Freshness), Ascorbic Acid, Asodicaronamide, Calcium Petroxide, Anylase Enzymes, Natural and Artificial Flavors (Contains Lemon), Colors (Annatto Extract, Titanium Dioxide, Turmeric). Contains wheat, soy, milk and eggs. Tree nuts may also be present in this product.

I'll just be straight up: YOU, WITH A SOY ALLERGY, STEP AWAY FROM THE HONEY BUNS —YOU MAY NOT EAT THIS! Seriously, this one's full of soy; let us count the ways: Soybean oil, yeast (maybe, especially if it's yeast extract), soy flour, soy lecithin, mono-diglycerides, glycerides, natural and artificial flavors. Plus we get the bonus label that tells us that this product is an allergen. There are alternatives that are soy free and just as delicious. Well, technically, no one should eat these, but we all have done, and continue to do. It's a classic.

CRISPY CRUST COMBINATION PIZZA:

This fast food style processed freezer pizza is a major NO-NO! We get the straight forward allergy labeling on this one.

- Ingredients: Enriched Flour (Wheat Flour, Malted Barley Flour, Niacin, Reduced Iron, Thiamine Mononitrate, Riboflavin, Folic Acid), Tomatoes (Water, Tomato Paste), Topping Blend (Mozzarella

Cheese Substitute[water, palm oil casein, modified food starch, non fat dry milk, sodium aluminum phosphate, lactic acid, sodium citrate, salt, potassium chloride, natural flavor, sorbic acid (as a preservative), artificial color, vitamin and mineral supplement (magnesium oxide, dicalcium phosphate, zinc oxide, riboflavin [Vitamin B2] electrolytic i4on, rolid qdie, pyridoxine hydrocholoride [Vitamin B6], niacinamide, thiamine mononitrate [Vitamin B1], syanocobalamin [Vitamin B12], Vitamin A palmitate]) Mozzarella Cheese [cultured pasteurized part skim milk, salt, enzymes]), water Fat Reduced Pepperoni (pork, mechanically separated pork, beef, water, textured vegetable protein product [Ingredients not in regular pepperoni] [soy protein concentrate, zinc oxide, niacinamid, ferrous sulfate, copper gluconate, Vitamin A palmitate, calcium pantothenate, thiamin mononitrate (B1), Salt, Containing 2% or less of spices, dextrose, lactic acid starter culture, oleoresin of paprika, flavoring, sodium nitrite, BHA, BHT, Citric Acid, Cooked Pizza Topping (Sausage [pork, mechanically separated chicken, spices, water, salt}]. Vegetable shortening (palm oil, butter flavor, soy lecithin). Yeast, contains 2% or less of sugar, vegetable oil (soybean, cottonseed, corn and/or canola oil), salt, modified food starch, paprika, spice, maltodextrin, isolated carrot product, citric acid, dough conditioner (wheat starch, L-Cysteine Hydrochloride, Ammonium Sulfate), onion, garlic, ascorbic acid. Contains:

142

wheat, milk and soy.

The giveaways are Textured Vegetable Protein (Soy Flour), and Soy Oil. Textured Vegetable Protein, as we now know, is one of the primary derivatives of the soybean, and the main source of the allergen. Definitely one to avoid on a soyfree diet. No one should eat this; it is junk food on general principles. Concentrate on more healthy food, allergy or otherwise.

HONEY GRAHAM STICKS:

This is a great snack offering from a natural food company; nice. Do they contain soy?

- Ingredients: Unbleached Wheat Flour, Evaporated Cane Juice, Safflower Oil, Graham Flour (Whole Grain Wheat Flour), Honey, Brown Rice Syrup, Leavening (Baking Soda, Monocalcium Phosphate), Sea Salt, Natural Flavor. Contains Wheat.

This would not be a safe product on a wheat free diet but for a soyfree diet it is safe. There are no soy products here; buy it and enjoy it. The only remote possibility for soy is in the Natural Flavor designation, but my family has used this product post allergy with no side effects whatsoever. It has a basic trust element on its side. This one would be worth contacting the manufacturer to find out the source of the natural flavor. Alright, I'll tell you the brand of this one; it's called Back to Nature Food Company.

RED BERRIES CEREAL:

A famous brand that everyone knows; let's look at it and determine if it has soy.:

- Ingredients: Rice, Whole Grain Wheat, Sugar, Wheat Bran, Freeze-dried Strawberries, Brown Sugar Syrup, Soluble Wheat Fiber. Contains 2% or less of salt, malt flavoring. Vitamins and minerals added: Vitamin C (ascorbic acid), reduced iron, Vitamin E (Alpha tocopherol-acetate), niacinamide, Vitamin B6 (Pyridoxine hydrochloride), Vitamin B1 (Thiamin hydrochloride), Vitamin B2 (riboflavin), Vitamin A palmitate, folic acid, Vitamin B12. Contains wheat ingredients.

This is basically safe and you can eat it and enjoy it. There is a potentially minute indicator with the tocopherol, but I'll refer you back to the earlier discussion about this derivative—Vitamin E (Tocopherol) can be soy based, but not always. If in doubt contact the manufacturer before buying.

GERMAN CHOCOLATE CAKE MIX:

Another famous brand of cake mix; this is a variety of chocolate cake, so you expect to see more in terms of flavorings and additives; how does it fare on soy?

- Ingredients: Sugar, Enriched Bleached Wheat Flour (Flour, Niacin, Reduced Iron, Thiamine Mononitrate, Riboflavin, folic Acid), Vegetable Oil shortening (Partially Hydrogenated Soybean Oil, Propylene glycol Mono- And Diesters Of Fats, Mono- And Diglycerides), Dextrose, Leavening (Sodium Bicarbonate, Dicalcium Phosphate, Sodium aluminum Phosphate, Monocalcium Phosphate), Cocoa Processed With Alkali. Contains 2% Or Less Of: Wheat Starch, Salt, Polyglycerol Esters Of Fatty Acids, Partially Hydrogenated Soybean Oil, Cellulose Gum, Xanthan Gum.

The vegetable oil in this mixture is composed of soybean oil, plus it has xanthan gum, which, as we know, we should be wary of; for these two elements, we shouldn't choose this one. Neither of these is required to be listed as an allergen, but they could represent the presence of soy, non-the-less. There is also a presence of mono-and diglycerides, which, as we know, could reveal hidden soy.

DAILY VITAMIN FOR MEN'S HEALTH:

I wanted to include this one to illustrate the widespread use of soy. This is a famous brand of dietary supplement/vitamin that I take everyday; it doesn't cause me any problems but for a soy allergy sufferer it's a major no-no. I wasn't aware that supplements and vitamins contained soy until I started the information gathering for the book. I was amazed at where I found soy hiding. This also points out clearly why you need to read labels. Let's read this label to see first hand the extent of soy:

- Dicalcium Phosphate, Calcium Carbonate, Magnesium Oxide, Microcrystalline Cellulose, Ascorbic Acid, Gelatin, Croscarmellose Sodium, di-Alpha Tocopherol Acetate, Stearic Acid, Calcium Silicate, Zinc Oxide, Niacinamid, Dextrin, Magnesium Stearate, Manganese Sulfate, Calcium Pantothenate, Pyridoxine Hydrochloride, Dextrose, Cupric Oxide, Riboflavin, Thiamin Mononitrate, Vitamin A Acetate, Lecithin, Sodium Cholecaiciferol, Cyanocobalamin, **Contains: Soy, Gluten Free**.

We get the required warning on this one. This one does contain soy, and wouldn't be indicated for a person with a soy allergy. This was perhaps one of the most interesting areas when I was reading and ferreting out information to put the guide together, and the most surprising. Who knew that a supplement would have soy? I've since learned that herbals, pharmaceuticals, vitamins, etc contain soy in a lot of forms: Powder for binding, oil, other oil derivatives for the coatings on pills and such. That's why you see the magnesium stearate listed in this vitamin. The magnesium stearate is what makes that smooth, slick covering on the pill.

Let's remind ourselves that the basic safety measure is to read the labels on everything so that you don't ever get caught by surprise, and innocently ingest something that passed under your radar. Since we're on the subject of pharmaceuticals here and the issue of where soy is, it's very important to remind your regular doctor at every opportunity so that he or she doesn't forget that you have the allergy because a large number of prescribed medicines have some form of soy as well.

In most cases, that soy presence will be in the coatings on pills as magnesium stearate, which is used to form an enteric coating that acts as a stomach buffer and creates a time release element. A lot of other soy products are present, such as lecithin, tocopherol-acetate, and other ingredients as binders. It's an area that doesn't get a lot of attention. We concentrate most of our effort on shoring up and safeguarding our food. It's very important that considering the nature of the allergen and its far flung presence, we need to take full stock of what we automatically use and what we take for granted.

NOTE ABOUT MONOSODIUM GLUTAMATE (MSG), AND YEAST:

MSG and Yeast are special considerations in relationship to soy, and bear some pull-out discussion. MSG and yeast, though technically not soy are connected by certain strands of chemical tinkering to the magic bean and to each other. In this context it is actually yeast extract that we're referencing; when reading labels, and determining what you can and can't eat, yeast extract and MSG need to be on your cautionary list. A long time ago, long before MSG became infamous and revealed as a useless and potentially dangerous food additive, MSG was manufactured from seaweed; its only use was and is as a flavor turbo-booster to a type of food called a savory, (umami)—it won't help your garden salad, but if added to meat, it'll cause you to drool. Presently, MSG is produced industrially in large mega-batches. There are a few ways of getting MSG: Hydrolysis (Extraction), Chemical Synthesis, and Fermentation. Glutamic acid, which makes up MSG and Yeast Extract, also occurs naturally and can point to a hidden soy connection through soy protein. When the constituents of the bean are unbound by chemical processing, the yield is amino acids and glutamic acid or MSG. Although MSG or yeast extract most likely won't cause a reaction, anyone with a soy allergy, actually everyone, would do well for their health and safety by not using any products with these useless—I'm sorry, I should say non-essential—ingredients. Finally, this product can be an associative allergen.

CHAPTER NINE
WHAT ABOUT MY FOOD BUDGET?

There will be some adjustments, and undeniably there will be some items that will be more expensive to buy and cook. The closer you get to totally fresh and whole foods, the more you will pay. The short answer is that it will be slightly more costly, but it won't be so out of reach that the average household or individual can't absorb it. There are also tradeoffs in certain areas of your food buying habits that will help you bring some balance.

Here's a baseline bit of advice to start us out: In the case of one allergy sufferer in the family, it would be advantageous on all fronts for the whole family to go as soyfree as possible; whereas there might be some added cost associated with this strategy, it would also eliminate the need for

150

double-batching, i.e., preparing one meal for the allergy sufferer and another for everyone else. That would get very expensive. You won't miss the soy, and might even feel better overall.

#

There are a lot of staples that won't change and it will be business as usual, and you will be able to plan your grocery shopping without much rearrangement. In some cases it might require you to make a few more stops to find items that you might not be able to find at your regular grocery store, but the larger outlets are more accommodating with a lot of variety; also you can count yourself fortunate if you live in a larger city because you are at a definite disadvantage if you live in a smaller town or rural community. Having an allergy in a rural setting would provide you the motivation to grow it yourself and at least have fresh garden foods available. That isn't to preclude the possibility of gardening in an urban setting, or even gardening inside. Gardening can be a rewarding thing.

Your main expense will be in fresh foods and specialty foods. Anything tagged as organic or natural will cost a little more. Here is a good point for me to make my position on organic more clear. My intention is not to imply that in order to be allergy free you have to go organic, although there is absolutely nothing wrong with it if that is your goal. That discussion calls for for full focus, and brings up possible directions for the future, but for now, suffice to say that allergy-free and organic are not synonymous, and 'organic' can be a questionable designator. For clarity, organic refers to how something is grown, and doesn't have anything to do with eliminating an allergen; the allergen can be present in organic products. Additionally, you could end up paying for hype without much return benefit in terms of nutrition and health.

#

A very important point is that you will need to work from your community level, and shop according to what's available in your local area. You will ultimately have to shop a little differently for some things that you need to accommodate your allergy. Certain things cost more anyway, such as processed foods, even the allergy friendly ones, and making things from scratch will ultimately cost less. That may seem counter intuitive on first pass.

You can always choose to go organic, keeping in mind the caveat above, but that will definitely cost you more, and that will only apply if you want to totally clean up your food act post allergy diagnosis. If you do decide to go organic, you can expect from that alone, to pay anywhere from, on the low end, $10 to even, on the high end, $50 more per month on your groceries. It's important to reiterate, though, that you don't have to buy only organic foods to eliminate the allergen from your diet.

Allergy friendly, or allergy aware, foods will also cost more, and foodstuffs such as specialty breads will realistically cost anywhere from $1.00 to even $3.00 more per loaf. You can work the details out in your own private space; you know your buying habits, and you know your budget. I won't insult anyone by presuming to set up some kind of budget that may not be applicable.

Ice cream can be upwards to $3.00 more per gallon if you're searching for soyfree or a specially made ice cream to accommodate another allergen. Mayonnaise, in this context, soyfree mayonnaise, is on the average almost $8.00 for a 24 oz. jar. Baking chocolate will cost more; expect to pay more for chocolate chips to use in baking.

There are several things you can do to keep from crashing your food budget.

- **Plan your meals carefully**
- **Buy some things in bulk; you can get discounts that way.**
- **Use coupons**—I used to be anti-coupon, but over time I've changed my thinking on that somewhat.
- **Look for special deals**
- **Shop online;** Amazon offers free shipping and subscription services on certain things. Of course, you can't order everything.
- **Buy the mass of your unaffected items in outlet stores** that naturally have lower prices. There's nothing wrong with these stores. Your mainstays and your staples for the most part won't be affected by the

allergy, and of course your fresh vegetables and fruits won't as well, and why not get these items from a source that will save you money. Don't be embarrassed to shop at outlet stores; you'll definitely get more for money spent.

- **Different companies will often offer deals if you join their mailing list.** If you have some favorite foods, go to the company websites and take advantage of any special offerings and deals they may have going as an incentive. As a consumer it is definitely advantageous for you to tag your favorite foods and provide feedback whenever and wherever you can. Be wary of your dealings with some companies, however, because some have begun enacting strange, shady policies that state that if you friend them, like them on social media, or sign up for any special deals on their site, you essentially lose the right to sue them for any damages they might cause with their manufacturing processes and corporate practices.
- **If you find a reliable source for soyfree items, stick with it:** Not only will you be able to predict cost more long-term, but you'll save time and money in other ways.
- **Buy the store brands:** The food is just as good, and you'll definitely save money on your trips to the grocery store.
- **Use social networking** to connect with

others for advice, tips and support.

A budget is based on household size, income, and other factors that can't all be covered in this limited scope. My aim isn't to attempt to spell it out for you, but to give an overview of how an allocated food budget might change with the allergen in the mix. This book is about managing your allergy, and taking a holistic approach is warranted, I think. The cost of groceries, food across the board, are rising constantly, and adding in extra-ordinary dietary needs can have a definite impact on your expenses. That mandates it be done with more sharply directed thought and stated purpose; if you are in the habit of going to the store without a list, it might be worth looking at changing that shopping pattern.

The greatest impact of the allergy is in the area of direct additives and proteins such as soy flour and isolates. Those are where you have to concentrate the most energy in eliminating and substituting. In line with that, it shouldn't come as a major surprise to see that this is where the core of the extra expense falls as well. You will find some refreshing and wonderful trade-offs in your shopping pilgrimage to replace soy. Fresh fish, for example, you will find to be much more economical and healthy for you and your family overall than those breaded, packaged varieties in the freezer section.

CHAPTER TEN
GENERAL EFFECTS
OF SOY

Here is what I'm not doing with this book: I'm not pointing an almighty judgmental finger; I'm not here to completely demonize soy; I'm not here to establish polarized camps of true belief; I'm not here to start any brand wars; I'm here to advocate for the best health and nutrition practices for us all. Should we eliminate soy from all our diets; that is probably not a reasonable course of action any more than consuming the mountain of the stuff that each of us consumes in a lifetime. There is, though, a middle path that we need to explore for our continued collective and individual health. Soy is undeniably a staple for millions of people the world over. With that stated, I will say that I'm a food activist; after reading and doing a great deal of research, I'm more and more developing a deep, and urgent desire to know what is going into what we eat on a daily basis. Ultimately, I'm not a die-hard soy fan either. I stated back in the introduction that soy is basically good, and I'll stick with that statement overall, but there is cause to think that soy isn't a miracle food as the masses have been and are being led to think. Soy is good with certain conditional factors.

For ongoing collection and summary, there are a few things I've learned about soy:

- Soy allergy is increasing in the developed world.
- Soy allergy has increased among infants and children.
- Soy products are not all created equal— fermented soy foodstuffs appear to be more beneficial and healthy than the highly manipulated protein.
- Soy protein is more of an allergen than the soy oil based products.
- There are some known and suspected problems with soy; all is not totally evil, but all is not perfect in soy world, either.
- Soy infant formula is probably not the best alternative for you baby.
- Soy isn't the great answer for women's health.
- Soy isn't the answer for men's health.
- Soy is subject to exposure to an inordinate amount of pesticides.
- Soy is a Genetically Modified Organism

(GMO).

- The upswing in soy allergy coincides with the introduction of genetically modified soybeans in 1994.

Soy is present in some form in over 30,000 products being manufactured at this point in history, both foodstuffs and industrial items. A rough estimate, and it's hard to visualize, puts the movement of soybeans from Argentina, Brazil and the United States at about 43 million tons per year. If you loaded all of those beans together into train cars, the train carrying them would wind around the earth over 1,000 times; about 1,041 times to be more exact. That is definitely a lot of soybeans. Where do those soybeans end up? They end up in our food supply; they end up in our animals' food supply; they end up in make up; they end up in toiletries; they end up in cleaning supplies; they end up in medicine and vitamins and supplements; they end up in just about any industry you can think of; in short, they end up in everything.

#

The soybean and its derivatives have been present in our food supply for many generations, and at this point a great deal is known about its positive and negative effects. Those who argue unequivocally for the positive benefits downplay soy's negatives for what it adds to those with special dietary needs and requirements. The purpose of this book isn't to make an absolute case against soy. However, I'll make no denials that after doing research into soy's effects as an allergen, I have some problems with soy's overall standing in our general food supply.

Soy has been studied and altered over the years with inventive and utilitarian results. We use soy derivatives daily that we can barely pronounce. We add some of the same products to both foodstuffs and household items. We add the same chemical concoctions to pharmaceuticals and cleaning products.

Undoubtedly there are many soy foods that are healthy, but there are some indications that all might not be perfect in soyland. My wife often says that the more she learns about soy, about the associative, reported effects and potential problems continually brought to light the more grateful she is that she has a soy allergy, and indeed looking closely at some of those problems helps us put the allergy into broader perspective and explains further how it became an allergen in the first place.

As I stated earlier, my goal isn't to totally denigrate soy or to turn soy into the arch-enemy legume, but I do want to look at all sides to give you, the allergy sufferer, a wider perspective. Plus, it is beginning to appear that everyone, allergy sufferers and non-allergy sufferers alike can benefit greatly without soy in their food or their life, or at the very least, a lot less of it.

So this chapter, then, is to focus on the positives that may come out of having the allergy

—what can someone with a hyper-sensitivity to a particular food teach us all about how to view our overall nutrition in a more conscious way?

The fact of the matter is we take food for granted! We make our inconvenient forays through the traffic and crowds down to our local grocery store chain with its great cornucopia of choices, and we start taking items off the shelves, tossing them into the cart and lug it all home. We rarely read labels, and we never stop to consider what those unpronounceable added things are and what they might be doing to our bodies and general health. A person with an allergy knows; she has to know. It's called conscious eating; it's called alert eating. This is the point where a hamburger bun could be potentially deadly because the soy flour that is most assuredly in it could bring about Anaphylaxis.

First of all, what does soy offer in terms of positive nutritional value? Soy's primary value is as a protein alternative, which is gold to vegans, vegetarians, and others who may have special dietary requirements, but that same protein is poison to people who are allergic to it. Soy is also prized as a filler because it expands the food supply and helps make food affordable and accessible to masses of people. That's certainly a laudable notion if some of that filler was added for more than—let's say—cosmetic effect. In some cases, soy is added merely to make food look more sleek and pretty. That, of course, is the wrong reason to add anything because that makes the additive unnecessary.

Everyone consumes a lot of soy everyday with no apparent ill effects, but is that reliable? Could there be cumulative results that show themselves years later. Is it possible to consume too much soy? There are some who think so, and there might be studies and research enough to support the notion that we should all wean ourselves from an over-reliance on soy, and remove it from our individual diet considerations and maybe from our food supply, but that latter is perhaps too radical a concept and maybe not doable, since it, meaning soy, is so ingrained.

There is one improvement that those in the circle of an allergy sufferer can make. They can take a cue from the focused attempts of the allergy sufferer to eat consciously, and become more connected to their own nourishment. This could be a major positive that comes out of wrestling with the allergy; it could represent a learning curve for everyone. It could mean that everyone changes their eating habits for the better. This chapter compares the benefits and hazards associated with having soy in our diets. We know what it means for someone with an allergy to avoid soy altogether, but should everyone eliminate soy or at least moderate the amount of it they consume? Let's find out.

Soy is billed as the cheapest source of protein, which ostensibly accounts for its widespread use as both a filler and as an alternative to animal protein. Soybeans can produce twice as much plant protein as any other crop and it is a complete protein. Soy is the number one protein replacement choice for vegans and vegetarians, and it is indeed jam-packed with protein and amino acids, making it the go to product for people with special diet requirements. Soy is low in calories. Soy is a great source of minerals, iron and vitamins, especially vitamin C.

As a viable protein, soy would be somewhere in the range of number five or six on a top ten list from nuts and seeds to the various meat products. It's easy to see that soy is a much sought after commodity both for the economics and the wide range of yield and applications. Reducing it to that, however, may not be the best way to look at a product that is so pervasive in our food supply, and that is supposed to nourish us without the civilized side effects.

There may, indeed, be side effects. There may, indeed, be harmful aspects to soy that all eaters need to be cognizant of, not just allergy sufferers. Now, the camps that laud soy for all its obvious benefits will not readily debate the pros and cons of a foodstuff that has taken the world by storm, and will, in most encounters, only champion the positives and gloss over the negatives. Why that is done is because pro-soy factions are about moving soy, increasing soy production, selling soy as is the way of everything; it's all about the economics and that makes perfect global sense. But as it is also about the supposed magic protein that may not always make good medical or nutritional sense. So, then, the double whammy of economics plus a readily available protein source makes soy hard to unseat from its lofty pedestal.

It's important, though, for all our benefit, to bring some balance to the discussion, and work from a level playing field. For a fair comparison let's look at some other possible negative effects that we should all be aware of. Soy allergy is only prevalent in developed countries. We'll start there, and work our way through the list of problems to arrive at a complete understanding of the great bean.

GENETIC MODIFICATION:

Did you know that the soybean is the first GMO or genetically modified organism? It is. The modification was to turbo-boost it so that it could withstand pesticides, in other words to ROUNDUP proof it. Glyphosate is the active chemical in ROUNDUP; between 180 to 200 million pounds are sprayed on lawns and agricultural crops every season. Soybeans are bombarded with more than the average amount of this herbicide; soybeans have the tendency to attract lots of weeds that can smother them out, and in order to protect them, growers spray inordinate amounts of pesticides on the crops, but the soybean, bolstered by its mutated genes, thrives while everything around it dies. GMOs are in the news, and rightfully so. There is definitely an ongoing need to know when it comes to figuring out the effects of GMOs on our food; in altering our food supply, are we consequently altering ourselves in a negative way? I believe it is a reasonable assumption that if a chemical is being showered on the plant, at some point that chemical will find its way into the plant. We're assured by those who are supposed to know that the processes of filtering, cleaning and rinsing remove all traces of pesticides from the plant, and further that no pesticides enter the plant, but questions remain. It calls for diligent activism on the part of every consumer so food producers and manufacturers of these potentially dangerous, life altering products know that we're watching.

PHYTOESTROGENS:
All new parents should carefully deliberate regarding any prescription for soy formula and exhaust all other possibilities before feeding their infant a soy based product. The rise in food allergies are primarily seen in children, and there is some belief that this is due to an increased use of soy formula. The problem is, or appears to be, the phytoestrogens which are naturally in soy. Phytoestrogens are natural estrogen compounds found in plants, and they are more potent in soybeans than other plant sources for whatever fascinating and mysterious reason. Too much soy can bring about endocrine imbalances in both male and female children. In the interest of neutrality, the debate is ongoing, and study of these potential effects continues, but there is

some evidence to suggest that it might pose a cumulative risk, and problems won't show up until years later. Pro-soy camps vehemently and categorically deny that any problems exist, and that is to be expected. By the same token, those camps have also not proven definitively that there isn't a problem. The worst thing we can do for all of us is to let things stay at an impasse.

ISOFLAVONES:

Before the volcano of protest erupts, let me explain that isoflavones are good, overall, but they can be bad. Isoflavones are connected to phytoestrogens discussed above, and a good balance is great, and certain sources suggest that they are very beneficial to women's health, helping to fight a number of female specific problems, fortification against the development of breast cancer, chiefly. But: the verdict is still out concerning what that balance is and how much is too much for optimum benefit. Other studies suggest that isoflavones may not be as friendly as regards men's health in terms of fighting prostate cancer. Also, there are indications that suggest isoflavones will actually reduce immune function. Furthermore, there are also findings from various sources that isoflavones can hasten the growth of cancer cells. All of these potential effects need diligent study, and while the verdict is still out, debate is a healthy thing.

PESTICIDES:

Pesticides are touched on in reference to GMOs, and in that case, ROUNDUP is the focus product. In this section, let's take a look at the negative associations with pesticides, and how they potentially affect our food and our health. Contrary to popular assertion to the contrary, pesticides do find their way into our food supply, and in reference to the soybean, you get a mega dose being poured onto the crop. The problem is that ROUNDUP only guarantees the crop won't be overrun, but there is nothing to guarantee that the pesticide won't find its way into the plant, and cause major systemic problems all the way down the line.

A fascinating thing to note is that a sharp rise in reported allergy to soy coincides with the introduction of modified soy into the food supply in 1994. The genetic modification as well as the pesticides could account for the upswing in sensitivity to soy protein. I want to be sure to reiterate that none of these assertions are proven beyond a shadow of a doubt: The FDA, and the Soybean Association assure us that soy is safe; those who see a problem with soy tell us that soy is an evil bean that will cause devastating cumulative problems. Meanwhile, the regular consumer continues to eat soy derivatives in mass quantities while factions of special interest argue over the quality and safety, but yet continue to up the production values purely for the economics. So what's the deal? The answer is that it isn't known for sure, and if soybean growers and producers know, they won't tell. Besides what has been mentioned above, these following are possibilities according to some:

- **Women's health**—while earlier touted by some camps as a super food with regard to helping fight breast cancer, there are some who think that ingesting too much soy can aggravate cancer, or speed up the growth of cancer cells.
- **Men's health**— factions believe that the excess amount of phytoestrogens in soy lead to male endocrine problems: erectile dysfunction, gynecomastia, (enlargement of breasts), as well as loss of libido, plus soy has zero positive effect on prostate health as has been asserted in other places.
- **Children's health**—the biggest possible consequence of an over-reliance on soy for children is endocrine imbalance, again those phytoestrogens, causing an early onset of puberty.
- **Aging**—there are some studies that suggest that those who rely on soy as a staple food product age faster than those who don't.
- **Imbalances**—it has been purported by some sources that overuse of soy leads to serious imbalances in certain key vitamins and minerals, namely zinc, iron and

calcium. That is because of the phytates. What are phytates? Also called phytic acid, phytates are antioxidants found in legumes and other plants that are known to bind to certain minerals so as to prevent their absorption into the system, leading to an imbalance. Over reliance on soy as a primary food can bring about this imbalance in key minerals and other nutrients. The Soyfoods Council disagrees with that assertion in their literature.

- **Gout**—For gout sufferers, or people with other forms of arthritis, consuming a lot of soy based foods may not be such a good idea.

- **Kidney Function**—it is possible that overuse of soy will cause kidney stones. The focus here is on a set of chemicals called oxalates; oxalates are the main components of kidney stones. Oxalates or oxalic acid are high oxidants that release what are called free radicals in your body, making it difficult to metabolize and eliminate these irritants from your body. Soy foods contain turbo-boosted levels of oxalates, which can, over time overload your system, creating the debilitating stones, and can also cause other damage to your body as well.

- **Thyroid function**—Hypothyroidism is the problem in this case. Overuse of soy can cause the thyroid to malfunction.

168

The magic word we see touted a lot is balance. Make sure you balance your diet, balance your calories, balance your diet with your activity level so that you don't gain weight—by the way, that's another potential problem with soy, creating weight gain. Well, there is one small problem with regard to that watchword; lest we forget, soy is being pumped into everything. With soy it is difficult to find a balance if the food producers and the soy peddlers insist on inundating us with soy.

The bottom line question becomes: Should you make an effort to be soy free? Well, ultimately it's a call for each person to make. With this book, I've tried to not paint soy as the monster food, and to be fair, soy is good in balance—there's that word again—but it's not so problem free that it should be considered a miracle food either. You will see factions stationed at each of these polarized points. The reality is somewhere in-between, where the rest of us live and eat. I've said that before; it bears repeating.

If, as a soy allergy sufferer, you want to encourage those in your wider circle to join you in being soy free, that is a noble cause. I'm working on doing so, and I haven't missed the soy. I still eat soy a little because I'm not allergic, but because my wife has the allergy, I will tell you that I read labels more carefully, I'm definitely more cognizant of what I put in my mouth, I'm actively concerned about my family as a whole, and more aware of what large food conglomerates are doing to our food supply in the cause of pure economics devoid of the element of caring. I don't think they, (they know who they are, those big monopolizers), care at all. There is a reason why the bulk of statistics and findings come with the qualifier: 'not definitive', 'not clearly established'; it's because the definitive answer isn't desired.

Is soy absolutely bad for you? I won't say that, but it can't hurt you to retake greater control over your diet, and perhaps limit your intake of such an overbearing foodstuff. You won't miss it; I don't. I also won't tell you that I've experienced this life altering change in my outlook, energy level or whatever; there could be unseen benefits that will only be apparent down the road. I will tell you this: it feels good to be conscious and more alert about food. I'm bothered by the notion that some conglomerate is trying to force feed me something because it's cheap and pads the corporate pocketbook.

You don't have to eat it just because it's on the grocery shelf or in the grocery freezer. Don't be fooled by all of the packaging and hype. Think of it as an adventure, a democratic experiment— food is more political than you think. Try it on for size; start to consciously think "less soy", start to consciously read labels, get familiar with some of those unpronounceable words, start to ask yourself, "should those things even be in my food at all?", educate yourself, and then explore for all of the wonderful alternatives that are out there.

Oh, yes, before I forget it, if you only do one thing, make one major change in the way you eat you can stop consuming that brand of 'stuff' we call 'fast' food. You don't need it, it costs too much, and besides all kinds of built in allergens like soy, it's pumped full of bad carbs, too much fat, and other non-nutrients that won't do anything for your health and well being except to make you overweight, bloated, and primed for a heart attack. There you are, I've said it, and the ball is now in your court.

CHAPTER ELEVEN
RESOURCES AND HELP

BIBLIOGRAPHY OF REFERENCE MATERIAL

Allergic Girl: Adventures in Living Well with Food Allergies, Sloane Miller

Allergy Guide: Alternative & Conventional Solutions (Smoots Guides), Elizabeth Smoots MD

Dealing with Food Allergies: A Practical Guide to Detecting Culprit Foods and Eating A Healthy, Enjoyable Diet, Janice Vickerstaff Joneja

The Everything Food Allergy Cookbook:

Prepare Easy-to-Make Meals Without Nuts, Milk, Wheat, Eggs, Fish or Soy, Linda Larsen

Food Allergies: A Complete Guide for Eating When Your Life Depends on It (A Johns Hopkins Press Health Book), Scott H. Sicherer, Hugh A. Sampson and Maria Laura Acebal

Food Allergies and Food Intolerance: The Complete Guide to Their Identification and Treatment, Jonathan Brostoff and Linda Gamlin

Food Allergies & Grandchildren: Pocket Guide for Grandparents (Allergy Free Table), Julie Trone

Food Allergies & Schools: Pocket Guide for Educators, Julie Trone and Maria Acebal

Food Allergy Handbook: A Quick-Start Survival Guide for People Learning to Eliminate Allergy Foods From Their Diets, Britt Boston

The Hidden Dangers of Soy, Dianne Greg

Hidden Food Allergies: The Essential Guide to Uncovering Hidden Food Allergies-and Achieving Permanent Relief, James Braley

Kids' Food Allergies for Dummies, Mimi Tang and Katie Allen

Natural Guide to Allergies (2nd Edition): From Pollen to Peanuts (Woodland Health), Louise Tenney

Natural Solutions for Food Allergies and Food Intolerances: Scientifically Proven Remedies for Food Sensitivities, Casey Adams, PhD. D.

Serving People with Food Allergies: Kitchen Management and Menu Creation, Schaefer and Joel J.

So, What Can I Eat?! Living Without Dairy, Soy, Eggs and Wheat, Rhonda Peters

The Unhealthy Truth: One Mother's Shocking Investigation into the Dangers of America's Food Supply, and What to Do about It, Robyn O'Brien and Rachel Kranz

The Whole Soy Story: The Dark Side of America's Favorite Health Food, Kaayla T. Daniel

Understanding Your Food Allergies and Intolerances: A Guide to Management and Treatment, Wayne Shreffler, Qian Yuan and Karen Asp

WEBSITES AND BLOGS

www.aafa.org: Asthma and Allergy Foundation of America (AAFA):

www.aap.org: American Academy of Pediatrics (AAP): A great source of information about infant and childhood allergies, infant formula and alternatives.

http://www.allerdine.com: Aller Dine: Aller Dine is a website that helps the diner find allergy friendly restaurants.

www.allergyeats.com: Allergy Eats: Allergy Eats is a website that provides a portal for finding allergy friendly restaurants.

www.allergicliving.com: Allergy Magazine covering food allergies as well as all the other allergens we're endlessly faced with.

www.acaai.org: American College of Allergy, Asthma, and Immunology, ACAAI. Professional articles on allergies, plus you can find an allergist in your local area.

www.nutrition.org: American Society for Nutritional Sciences; a portal for food allergy information as well as other food issues regarding nutrition labeling standards.

http://www.cehn.org/center evaluation risks hu man reproduction cerhr: Center for the Evaluation of Risk to Human Reproduction (CERHR): More information on soy infant formula.

www.crops.org: Crop Science Society of America; even though it's pro-soy for the most part, the myths on the history of soy are fascinating.

www.mercola.com: Dr. Mercola: Dr. Mercola is a food activist and a major force in finding what's in our food and how it might be harming us.

www.fda.gov: Food and Drug Administration (FDA): Find important information on food labeling and gain knowledge about legislation regarding our food supply.

www.foodallergy.org: FARE—Food Allergy Research and Education: Source of great information about how to manage food allergies— covers the top eight, including soy.

www.gmo-compass.org: GMO Compass: A site dedicated to keeping the public abreast of GMO issues.

www.hc-sc.gc.ca: Health Canada is the official health care site. It has many great resources and in depth information on food allergies.

www.jama.jamanetwork.com: Journal of the American Medical Association (JAMA):

www.jn.nutrition.org: Journal of Nutrition, published by the American Society of Nutrition. It's a great educational resource for food allergies.

www.kidshealth.org: Kid's Health.org is a wonderful site to go to for advice and information for babies, toddlers and teens.

www.livestrong.com: Livestrong.com. This is a vast site with much medical, nutritional, and allergy related information.

www.mayoclinic.org: Mayo Clinic has much educational information for food allergy sufferers.

www.msds.com: MSDS—Material Safety Data Sheet; MSDS is the go to source to find relevant information on any chemical substance in existence.

http://www.niehs.nih.gov: National Institute of Environmental Health Sciences (NIEHS): Of major interest here is the National Toxicology Program study on soy infant formula.

www.nih.gov: National Institute of Health (NIH): Find information and publications on allergies and other medical concerns.

www.nexusmagazine.com: Nexus Magazine is an alternative magazine on health and other issues. I discovered interesting articles on soy allergy, and soybeans from the site. With most articles, they want you to pay to read.

www.soyfoods.org: Soyfoods Association of North America; pro-soy but educational none-the-less.

www.thesoyfoodscouncil.com: Soyfoods Council is affiliated with Iowa Soybeans Association. Great defender of soybeans; it helps to look at all perspectives.

www.soyinfocenter.com: Quite an interesting and comprehensive history of soy from the soy industry side. A good source for information on soy and its presence in our food supply. It's pro-soy, of course, but it doesn't hurt to arm yourself with as much information as possible to help you manage your soy allergy.

www.uchicagokidshospital.org: Univ. of Chicago Comer Children's Hospital: lots of very accessible information on food allergy management for children and setting up a diet of allergy friendly foods.

https://www.facebook.com/foodallergiesonabudget: Food Allergies on a Budget: Social media connection; this is a group on Facebook that offers helpful tips and advice so that people can get the most out of their food dollar.

www.webmd.com: Web MD: Great storehouse of reliable information on any number of medical issues. The information on food allergies is educational and thorough.

SOURCES FOR SOYFREE FOOD

www.amazon.com: Amazon: Yes! Amazon is a good source for a large variety of specialty foods that can help you manage your food allergy.

www.amys.com: Amys has many possibilities for soy allergy sufferers; the site has an internal search tool that allows you to narrow your subject matter.

www.annies.com: Annie's Homegrown: Might be a little pricey for some, but Annie's is available at many grocery outlets.

http://www.bumblebee.com/: Bumblebee: Not all of the Bumblebee products are soyfree; there are a few items, but read labels carefully before you buy.

http://www.edwardandsons.com: Edward and Sons: A wonderful source for a wide variety of foods that are produced for the requirements of special diets; Lots of offerings for dealing with all food allergens, including soy. You may have to order products online; they're not available in many locations.

www.enjoylifefoods.com: Enjoy Life: Look for them in the specialty sections of your grocery store.

www.imaginefoods.com: Imagine has limited products in the areas of gravies, broths and sauces, but they're organic and free of the usual additives. Good for cooking with.

www.jiffymix.com: Jiffy: An interesting company that has been around awhile, and surprisingly there are a few soy free offerings, and the good news is that the brand is available at virtually every grocery store. The corn muffin and buttermilk biscuit mixes are good, (soyfree).

www.kitchenbasics.net: Kitchen Basics:

www.librenaturals.com: No Nuttin/Libre Naturals:

www.naturespath.com: Nature's Path:

http://oceannaturals.com/: Ocean Naturals Tuna: A good brand of tuna without soy additives.

www.oetker.ca: Dr. Oetker Organics:

www.pacificfoods.com: Pacific:

www.panerabread.com: Panera Bread: Panera isn't necessarily allergy friendly, and you need to ask questions. A few products are soy free.

www.rudisbakery.com: Rudi's Organic

www.shopwell.com: Nutritional information on scores of products; read labels, compare foods, and learn what foods are best for you and your dietary needs. A highly recommended site.

www.soyalternatives.com: The Kitchen: source for information, recipes for soy-free cooking and substitutions.

http://www.soyfreesales.com: Soy Free products from Oregon; offerings like chocolate, other candies, gourmet mixes, and yes, soy free gum.

www.traderjoes.com: Trader Joe's:

http://www.wildplanetfoods.com: Wild Planet:

ANAPHYLAXIS

Sites for information on auto injectors for administering epinephrine.

http://adrenaclick.com: Adrenaclick: Amedra

Pharmaceuticals, LLC

www.allerject.ca: Allerject: Sanofi-Aventis Canada; for Canadian Residents only.

www.anapen.co.uk: Anapen: Anapen is available primarily for the UK.

www.auvi-q.com:
Auvi-Q: Auvi-Q is the U.S. Version of the Allerject pen offered in Canada by Sanofi-Aventis.

www.emerade.com:
Emerade: Developed by Namtall/Medeca Pharma AB, Emerade is available for countries in Europe including Sweden, Norway, Finland, Denmark, UK, and Germany.

http://www.epipen.com: EpiPen, a product of Mylan, Inc, Mylan Specialty L.P.

www.jext.co.uk: Jext: A product of ALK-abelo Ltd in the UK.

FOOD ALLERGY LABELING REQUIREMENTS

Go to the FDA site and print out a copy of the allergy labeling law:
- Food Allergen Labeling and Consumer Protection Act of 2004

FALCPA:
http://www.fda.gov/Food/GuidanceRegulation/G
uidanceDocumentsRegulatoryInformation/Allerge
ns/ucm106187.htm

FDA Reportable Food Registry:
http://www.fda.gov/Food/ComplianceEnforceme
nt/RFR/default.htm#who
This is an industry compliance site, but is a good
site to visit to get a perspective on how issues are
handled through regulatory channels.

MEDIC ALERT IDENTIFICATION

www.AmericanMedical-ID.com:

www.oneidamedicaljewelry.com:

www.mediband.us:

www.medicalert.org:

www.medids.com:

www.n-styleid.com:

This is a sampling; explore to find more sources
for your needs.

CHAPTER TWELVE
MYTHS AND FACTS

I wanted to set up this last chapter as a series of myth versus fact statements in order to provide a summary of key points that were covered in the book, and perhaps draw out what might be important to remember beyond the cardinal rules for management that were laid out early on. You can call these highlights, talking points, maybe, so that you can be armed with certain knowledge bits to field any questions that are thrown at you. Many folks don't know about these things, and you can help them by being a knowledgeable advocate for safe nourishment. Most take it for granted, doing nothing more than rushing to the grocery store and loading up the cart with what they like, getting in a line, paying for it, and going home. All need to be better educated about our world, and the world of food is or should be no less a consideration; so while you're dealing with your allergy, you can be an educator. Enough of my preaching, go out, live well, eat well, know that you can deal with it, and you can eat safely and well.

MYTH: Only babies develop soy allergy.

FACT: People can develop soy allergy at any age. However, the recent sharp spikes in reported food allergies are among infants and children.

MYTH: Soy allergy is rare.

FACT: Most studies give a 1.0% estimate for the prevalence of soy allergy; although no truly definitive studies have been done that can pinpoint an exact figure, using that estimate alone would yield a result that gives pause. For example: If you start with one million people, and if you take the 1.0% as a benchmark, you will see that out of that 1,000,000, 10,000 people are affected by a soy allergen. That adds up to a lot of people who are directly affected by a simple food product. We also can't overlook the fact that soy is among the top eight food allergies.

MYTH: Babies will outgrow an allergy to soy.

FACT: Although there is some evidence to support the assertion, the verdict is still largely out, and anyone who has displayed sensitivity to a certain food will continue to display sensitivity and intolerance to some degree. The fact is that some babies will outgrow their allergy, but not all.

MYTH: Soy allergy only comes from food.
FACT: Soy is present in so many products that we use everyday that anyone allergic to soy can absorb it through the skin by using topical products such as soaps, shampoos, lotions, etc. that may contain, and often does contain, soy derivatives. It is very important to read labels and know what you are putting in and on your body. For full disclosure, there is no clear proof that an allergen is absorbed through the skin by using derivative products, but the person with an allergy needs to possibly err on the side of the worst case scenario so as to remain safe.

MYTH: You can't eat well with a soy allergy.
FACT: It is true that the presence of soy and all of its variants in our food is mind-boggling in scope, and whereas it is difficult to find a grocery or restaurant item that doesn't contain soy in some fashion, it is possible to eliminate soy from your diet with a little bit of research and due diligence. There is life after the development of a soy allergy, and it is possible to eat well, and enjoy great tasting food without soy. You have to dial back the clock to a more simple time and develop a more basic mindset with regard to food—think raw, think fresh, think simple, think natural, think un-processed, think no additives, and think more direct involvement in food preparation.

MYTH: Soy protein is a naturally healthy food.
FACT: Soy is undeniably a great food in so many respects, and has added greatly to our food supply. Tofu, soy milk, and soy yogurt have become staples in the natural foodie world. All in all it is a highly beneficial product, but according to studies there are some recognized problems associated with soy protein; one such problem is that with long term use, soy can overload the pancreas and is a potential carcinogen. This determination is not firmly established, and it would be unfair to state that as an absolute finding. That is, however, concerning enough and should give us all pause.

MYTH: A food allergy is the same for all cases.
FACT: The symptoms can vary from mild to severe; one person's soy allergy isn't the same for the next person. A life-threatening situation for one will be a minor rash to another: That is why education is important; that is why knowing your body's tolerance levels and your personal limits are important.

MYTH: If you have an allergy to a certain food, you can never eat that food again.
FACT: An onset can be keyed to the amount you ingest; a teaspoonful of something may or may not cause a reaction, but three tablespoons will. One tiny drop may, but a whole plateful may not; it's unpredictable, and it just depends—on a lot of factors. Additionally, some by-products may or

may not be allergenic: Soy oil, diglycerides, lecithin, mono-diglycerides, vitamin E, (tocopherol acetate), for example. That is why you always need to avoid something that you have doubts about.

MYTH: If you are allergic to one food, you won't be allergic to others.
FACT: You can be allergic to more than one food; in the case of soy, if you are allergic to one legume you can be allergic to another in the same family which includes peanuts, lentils, and indeed all beans.

MYTH: You will know when you've been exposed to an allergen because the symptoms will appear instantly.
FACT: There is an odd phenomenon related to food allergies: The reaction can be delayed up to seventy-two hours, so the allergen contaminated food you ate on Thursday could make your weekend hell. There isn't any clear determination what causes this delayed reaction, and that makes being prepared for any surprises a major factor in food allergy management: Always have countermeasures with you—Benedryl, adrenaline injectors, something to sooth itching.

MYTH: Allergy shots will cure your allergy.
FACT: Allergy shots can be helpful in alleviating the effects of certain types of allergies, especially environmental allergies like dust, pollen, etc. but

there isn't any proof that allergy shots help with food allergies, and will at most only serve to mask symptoms for a period of time. There is no cure for food allergy, and expensive shots are a waste of time and money for a result that has virtually zero efficacy.

MYTH: If you have a problem with a food, it means that you are allergic to it.
FACT: An allergy and intolerance/sensitivity to a food are different. An allergen is defined as an irritant that affects the whole body, the immune system; an intolerance to a food in concentrated in the digestive, gastric system. Those problems can be caused by a sensitivity to a food or to food poisoning, or ingesting too much of a certain food. The total percentage of people who are affected by food allergies is 2% while some sources cite as much as 5%.

MYTH: The presence of hives are a sign of a food allergy.
FACT: Although hives commonly accompany other symptoms of an allergy attack, they are also present in a lot of other instances as well, so hives alone aren't a reliable indicator of an allergy. Hives can be present in drug reactions, insect bites, heat, cold or during infections.

MYTH: Food labeling requirements help people shop safely, and clear up confusion surrounding what's in food.

FACT: Food labeling requirements are helpful to a degree, but they by no means remove the need to be diligent about learning the different names of additives and components, and making sure that there aren't any hidden products in the food you are about to purchase. You will find mostly reliable information—if only the fulfillment of minimal requirements—about the eight major allergens, but they aren't the only allergy causing products by any means. In terms of soy, there are many products that are derived from soy that you need to know about, but that aren't required to be labeled as such, and other ingredients are exempt from the labeling laws, such as lecithin, and soy oil. Nothing beats your own research and self education so that you can go to the grocery store armed with the full knowledge you need to shop with confidence and make wise choices for your health and safety. No one knows your allergy better than you.

MYTH: If I take BENEDRYL before I go out, it will stop an onset even if I accidentally ingest the allergen.
FACT: It couldn't hurt to have the antihistamine in your system, and it would certainly help with the minor irritants of an eventual reaction, but it wouldn't protect you from a full blown reaction that could lead to anaphylactic shock. Plus it may not be wise to rely on a preemptive medicine to get you through; it might cause you to make risky choices. The better course might be a proactive

approach so that you can better control and react as necessary to your environment for you safety and health. You do, however, need to remember to carry allergy medication as well as your epinephrine with you at all times.

MYTH: There isn't anything to suggest that the mother will introduce an allergen in utero or by way of breast feeding.
FACT: There are some results from studies that bear findings to the opposite; in fact, early studies show that the baby while still in the womb can develop antibodies against soy protein; as well, the infant can also react to allergens through breast milk. It is important for parents, and for mothers who breast feed to be aware of this possibility so they don't expose their baby to a potential allergen. The general advice offered to new mothers is to reduce the amount of legumes such as soybeans and peanuts in their diet during the final stages of pregnancy. There is also a trend for new parents to seek alternatives to soy formula arising out of studies that show soy based products may not be the best choices for baby's nutrition.

APPENDICES

- ALPHABETIC LIST
  OF SOY PRODUCTS
- ALPHABETIC LIST OF FOOD
  & INDUSTRIAL ELEMENTS
  CONTAINING SOY
- LABEL READING GUIDE

SOY LIST

Here is a recap list of soy ingredients that you will see on labels of foods and household items. It will help you speed up your trips to the grocery store and streamline your food choices; eventually you won't need it, but it's a good rundown of items to look for to make shopping for soy-free items easier and less stressful. The list includes ingredients found in foodstuffs, topical, cosmetic and all manner of industrial products. A couple of simple reminders as you shop and make your decisions about what you should avoid: first, the Food and Drug Administration, (FDA), doesn't consider oil or its derivatives as allergens, but you know your allergy trigger points, and you should always make your choices carefully, refusing any food or other item that you think might be unsafe; second, pay extra attention to the items on the list that can reveal hidden soy as this is the area where you could ingest the allergen without knowing it.

Always read labels; manufacturers will at times change ingredients, adding the allergen, then removing it, creating circumstances where a food you could tolerate is no longer on your safe list, and a food you couldn't tolerate is now clear of the allergen and is therefore something you can safely eat. Remember that soy is everywhere; don't allow yourself to become complacent.

ALPHABETIC LIST
SOYBEAN FOODS, SOY-BASED
PRODUCTS AND SOY DERIVATIVES

A
Abura-age
Akara
Alkyl Chlorides
Alkyd Resin Solution
Artificial flavorings
Ascobyl Palmitate
Atsu-age

B
Bulking agent

C
Calcium caseinate
Caprylic Triglyceride
Carob
Cheonggukjang
Chunjang

D
Defoaming agent
Dimethylsoya
   Ammonium
   Ethosulfate
Doenjang
Doubanjiang
Douchi

E
Edamame
Emulsifier
Ethyldimethylsoya Alkyl
Et Soyethyldimonium
   Ethosulfate
Ethyl Sulfates

F
Fermented bean paste
Fish sauce

G
Gan-modoki
Gelatin
Gen'en
Glycine Max
Glycols
Gochujang
Guar gum

H
Honjozo
Hydrolized plant
   protein
Hydrolized soy protein
Hydrolized vegetable

protein
Hyojun

I

Infant formula (soy
 based)
Isolated vegetable
 protein
Isostearyl Isosterate

J

Jokyu
Joseon ganjang

K

Kecapasin
Kekap
Kekap manis
Kekap manis sedang
Kinako
Koikuchi
Kongo
Kongo-jozo
Kyodofu

L

Lecithin
Licorice

M

Magnesium stearate

Methylcellulose
Miso
Mono-diglyceride
Monosodium glutamate
 (MSG)
Mono-triglyceride
Morpholinium
 Compounds

N

Natto
Natural flavorings
Nimame

O

Okara
Olean
Olestra
Oyster sauce

P

Phospholipids
Phthalic Anhydride
Pickled tofu
Pinyin (Fermented Tofu)
Pinyin (stinky)
 (Fermented Tofu)
Polyethylene glycol
Polymer with
 Pentaerythritol
Protein
Protein extender

Protein Isolate

Q

Quaternary Ammonium
 compounds
Quaternary ammonium
 salts
Quaternium-9

S

Saishikomi
Shiro
Shoyu
Shrimp soy sauce
Soja
Sorbitan tristearate
Soya
Soya chunks
Soyatrimonium
 Chloride
Soy
Soyaethyl
Morpholinium
 Ethosulfate
Soy albumin
Soybean curd
Soybean granules
Soy fiber
Soy flour

Soy grits
Soy meat
Soy milk
Soy molasses
Soy nuts
Soy oil
Soy panthenol
Soy protein
Soy protein concentrate
Soy protein isolate
Soy Sauce
Soy sprouts
Soy sterols
 PEG 5
 PEG 10
 PEG 16
 PEG 25
 PEG 30
 PEG 40
Stabilizer
Starch
Stearic acid
Styrene
Supro
Sweet bean sauce

T

Tamari
Tauco
Tauchu
Tempeh
Teriyaki

Textured vegetable protein (TVP)
Thickener
Tianmianjiang (Sweet bean sauce)
Tocopherol-acetate
Tocotretrienols
Tofu
Tokkyu
Toyo
Trimethylsoya
Tuong
Tyramine

U

Unohana
Usujio
Usukuchi

V

Vegetable broth
Vegetable gum
Vegetable protein
Vegetable starch
Vegetable stearic acid
Vinyltoluene
Vitamin E

W

Worcestershire sauce

X

xanthan gum

Y

Yakidofu
Yeast extract
Yellow soybean paste
Yuba

Z

Zanthan gum

ALPHABETIC LIST
OF DIFFERENT PRODUCTS
THAT CONTAIN SOY ELEMENTS

SOY PROTEIN
FOOD PRODUCTS

ale
aquaculture *(the raising and harvesting of fish and other animals and plants in water)*
bread
baby food
bakery ingredient
beer
bee food
calf milk replacers
cake frosting
candy
candy ingredient
cereals
confection
cookie ingredient
cookie topping
cracker ingredient
doughnuts
dietary items
drinks
dairy feed *(soybean hulls)*
frozen desserts

fountain topping
fish foods
fox and mink feeds
green soybeans
grits
high fiber bread *(soybean hulls)*
hypo-allergenic milk
infant milk drinks
meat substitute
meat products
miso
natto
noodles
okara
pancake flour
pan grease extender
pet food
pie crust
poultry feeds
prepared mixes
protein concentrates
sausage casings
shaped pasta doughs
soy coffee
soy milk
soynut butter
soy nuts
soy sauce
special diet foods
stock feeds
sweet goods
swine feeds

tempeh
tofu
yeast

SOY OIL
FOOD PRODUCTS

bakery products
chocolate coatings
coffee whiteners
cookies
cooking oils
crackers
creamers
dietary
emulsifying agent
fatty acids
filled milk (*skim or condensed milk
with vegetable oil
added to replace fat content*)
glycerol *(sugar alcohol)*
liquid shortening
margarines
mayonnaise
medicines
pharmaceuticals
refined soybean oil
salad dressings
salad oils
sandwich spreads
shortening

snack foods
soy lecithin
stabilizing agent
sterols
supplements
vegetable shortening

SOY PROTEIN
INDUSTRIAL PRODUCTS

adhesive
analytical reagents
antibiotics
asphalt emulsions
binders *(wood/resin)*
cleansing materials
cosmetics
fermentation aids
fermentation nutrients
films for packaging
filter material *(soybean hulls)*
fungicides
inks
insecticidal sprays
leather substitutes
linoleum backing
livestock feeds
paints *(water based)*
particle board
pesticides
pharmaceuticals

plastics
plywood
polyesters
tape joint cements
textiles
texture paints
wallboard

SOY OIL
INDUSTRIAL PRODUCTS

anti-corrosive agents
anti-static agents
alcohol manufacture--
(antifoaming agents)
calf milk replacers
caulking compounds
core oils
cosmetics
diesel fuel
disinfectants
dust control agent
detergents
dispersing agent
electrical insulation
epoxies
fungucides
herbicides
inks *(printing inks)*
insecticides
linoleum backing

metal casting
metal work
margarine manufacture
(antispattering agent)
oiled fabrics
paints
pesticides
plasticizers
protective coatings
putty
shampoo
soaps
vinyl plastics
waterproof cement
wallboard
wetting agents
yeast manufacture

LABEL READING QUICK GUIDE

SOY PROTEIN

Soy protein is the main culprit. Avoid soy proteins at all cost. Don't use a product if you see these on the label:

Soy Flour • Textured Soy Flour (TSF) • Textured Soy Protein (TSP) • Textured Vegetable Protein (TVP) • Isolate • Diglycerides • Mono-diglyceride • Hydrolized Vegetable Protein (HVP) • Hydrolized Soy Protein (HSP) • Hydrolized Plant Protein • Edamame • Kinnoko Flour • Kyodofu • Miso • Soy Miso • Natto • Okara • Shoyu Sauce • Soy Albumin • Soy Bran • Soy Concentrate • Soy Fiber • Soy Grits • Soy Milk • Soy Nuts • Soy Nut Butter • Soy Sauce • Soy Sprouts • Soya • Soya Flour • Soybean Granules • Soybean Curds • Soybean Flour • Soybean Paste • Supro • Tamari • Tempeh • Teriyaki Sauce • Tofu • Yakidofu • Yuba • Protein Extender • Glycine Max •

SOY OIL

Products manufactured with soy oil are not as allergenic as soy protein products, but the food industry doesn't provide any guarantees that the manufacturing process rids the oil of all traces of proteins which may bring on a reaction; always ally yourself on the side of extreme caution:

Soy Oil • Vegetable Oil • Lecithin • Soy Lecithin •

OTHER SOURCES OR INDICATORS OF SOY

Artificial Flavorings • Natural Flavorings • Guar Gum • Xanthan Gum/Zanthan Gum • Vegetable Gum • Vegetable Broth • Vegetable Starch • Asian • Asian Foods • Chinese • Japanese • Thai • Vitamin E (Tocopherol Acetate) • Monosodium Glutamate (MSG) • Yeast • Yeast Extract • Emulsifier • Thickener • Polyethylene Glycol • Bulking Agent •

LABEL DESIGNATORS

Contains (this one is required if the product directly contains the allergen protein) • **May Contain** (this one is voluntary for the manufacturer, but you will see it included on labels fairly regularly) • **And/Or** (this is seen in relation to oil additives "...one or more of the following, canola and/or soy oil") • **Cross contamination warning** isn't required, but you will see it on labels quite often.

RULES

1) Always Read Labels **2)** If in Doubt, Avoid It **3)** Educate yourself **4)** Ask Questions, get Answers **5)** Contact the Manufacturers

---

INDEX

COLOPHON

Proudly self-published

WRITING AND MANUSCRIPT BUILDING
Manuscript preparation: Open Office Apache
Type
- Body text: Bookman Old Style, 12 pt.
- Internal text: Cambria, 12 pt.
- Headers: Bookman Old Style, 12 pt., 18 pt.
- Chapter titles: Bookman Old Style, 22 pt.
- Lists: Bookman Old Style, 12 pt.
- Other: Elephant, 26 pt.

PRE-PUBLICATION
Copy-editing/Proofreading: Bill Bowling, Katrina
Bowling, Anahlisha Bowling

COVER
Design: Anahlisha Bowling
Illustrations: Anahlisha Bowling

BOOK DESIGN
Book Design: Bill Bowling

FILE CONVERSION
Open Office Apache to PDF

PRINTING
Print on Demand
Paper: 60# white offset book
Cover: 10 pt C1S, four color, layflat film lamination
Binding: Perfect bound (adhesive, softcover)

ABOUT BILL

Bill Bowling is a writer, artist and teacher who has written both fiction and nonfiction; he is also a copywriter, and has produced operations documents and training manuals for businesses and start-ups in the Human Services field. Bill is also a poet who has published his first book of poetry entitled Perturbance: Flash Journal, The Sevenlings. His interest in writing about food allergies was sparked by the challenges his wife faced in managing a sudden onset allergy to soy. This first entry in the Food Allergy Guide Series is the result of shared experience along with much information gathering and research. Bill has a master's degree in Education, and has an active interest in the arts and arts education. He loves nature and walking around freely in the great outdoors. He lives in Kentucky surrounded by friends and family. You can make contact with Bill through Facebook, Twitter, G+, and Linked in. You can find his published works in poetry, fiction, nonfiction and other educational content on his website at www.billbowling.weebly.com, Amazon.com, and many other places where good books are sold. The most important thing is the writing and the basic reward in it; in that light, Bill works in different genres and from many interests. From the writer's perspective, a writer writes, period, and there shouldn't be any other conditional equations. Bill is also an avid reader and you will find him on Goodreads as well.

ORDER INFORMATION

TO FIND OUT MORE about the Guide to Soy, or to stay in the loop about future volumes of the FOOD ALLERGY GUIDE series, I invite you to visit the websites to say hi, sign up for special notifications and see what I've got going on: http://www.billbowling.weebly.com -Or- http://www.ridgelinepublishing.weebly.com

You can also connect on social media, Facebook, Twitter, G+, where you will find regular announcements and updates as well. I'm sure to see you out there somewhere. I'm very likeable, and I promise I don't bite.

If you would like to purchase more copies of THE FOOD ALLERGY GUIDE TO SOY, you can visit Amazon.com, or other outlets, nationally and internationally, where great books are sold.

If you would like to discuss bulk orders, contact me and I'll see what I can do for you.

Thank you for your purchase, and I look forward to hearing from you soon with your feedback about your experience with the book. I welcome suggestions on how I can improve my work.

Bill Bowling

COMING SOON . . .

Next Installment of the Food Allergy Guide Series:

• Food Allergy Guide to Peanuts

The FOOD ALLERGY GUIDE TO PEANUTS is the second volume in the series, and will cover in-depth this other famous legume with the definite misnomer—it isn't a nut. It starts there and unwinds to provide a guide for dealing with this number one allergen of childhood.

I invite you to sign up to receive notice of when this volume will be available. Details are also being worked out for pre-release deals; look for those details and get in the early bird line.

Http://www.billbowling.weebly.com

Thank you, good health and blessings to all.

. . . STAY TUNED

COMING SOON ...

The Companion Cookbook for Soy Allergies. A wonderful, delicious variety developed by a cook with a soy allergy:

- ## Muffin Kupp Kitchen Cookbook: Soy Free Recipes.
Recipes Created by Trina B.
Compiled and Organized
by Bill and Anahlisha Bowling

It's being assembled as fast as the little elves can work and will be ready soon. Oh, yes!

Muffin Kupp Kitchen is Trina B's blog. She's hinted that you can get a free recipe or two, plus find other gems of general and special interest. Sign up to be notified of release date and get in line for some nice surprises.

http://www.muffinkuppkitchen.com
http://www.billbowling.weebly.com

... STAY TUNED

NOTES:

MY FRIENDLY FOOD LIST

*Don't take anything for granted—read those
labels every time.

Made in the USA
San Bernardino, CA
26 February 2015